MW01293311

Exposing Bad Plastic Surgery

EXPOSING BAD PLASTIC SURGERY

and the SECRET to AVOIDING IT

- - - - - - - - - - - - -

Dr. Thomas J. Francel, FACS

NEW YORK

LONDON • NASHVILLE • MELBOURNE • VANCOUVER

EXPOSING *BAD* PLASTIC SURGERY

And the Secret to Avoiding It

© 2025 Dr. Thomas J. Francel, FACS

All rights reserved. No portion of this book may be reproduced, stored in a retrieval system, or transmitted in any form or by any means—electronic, mechanical, photocopy, recording, scanning, or other—except for brief quotations in critical reviews or articles, without the prior written permission of the publisher.

Published in New York, New York, by Morgan James Publishing. Morgan James is a trademark of Morgan James, LLC. www.MorganJamesPublishing.com

A portion of the proceeds from this book will be donated to the Arts as Healing Foundation in St. Louis. This charitable organization provides free art instruction to lower and middle-income women with cancer and other chronic illness. These classes represent a safe haven where patient-artists can forget their illness as they explore their artistic talents, collaborate with others, and gain relief from the stress and fear associated with their disease.

Proudly distributed by Publishers Group West®

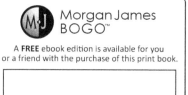

Morgan James BOGO™

A **FREE** ebook edition is available for you or a friend with the purchase of this print book.

CLEARLY SIGN YOUR NAME ABOVE

Instructions to claim your free ebook edition:
1. Visit MorganJamesBOGO.com
2. Sign your name CLEARLY in the space above
3. Complete the form and submit a photo of this entire page
4. You or your friend can download the ebook to your preferred device

ISBN 9781636984346 paperback
ISBN 9781636984353 ebook
Library of Congress Control Number: 2024932247

Interior Design by:
Chris Treccani | www.3dogcreative.net

Cover Drawings by:
Mary Lynn Brophy | MLBGraphic

Freehand Drawings by:
Terry Hinkle/Hinkle Creative
Instagram: @hinklecreative

Anatomical Drawings by:
Vicki Freidman

Photographs by:
Suzy Gorman | Suzy Gorman Photography

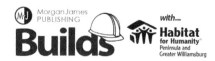

Morgan James PUBLISHING Builds with... **Habitat for Humanity** Peninsula and Greater Williamsburg

Morgan James is a proud partner of Habitat for Humanity Peninsula and Greater Williamsburg. Partners in building since 2006.

Get involved today! Visit: www.morgan-james-publishing.com/giving-back

To Marilyn, the love of my life, who claims she spent as much time editing as I did writing this book; my daughter Katya, who also helped to edit the manuscript as well as serve as our model for Natural and Aesthetic Ideals; and my sons, Nicholas and Michael, who spent many years "fatherless" as I completed my general surgery and plastic surgery training.

Contents

A Note to the Reader

This book contains descriptions of surgical procedures and images that may be considered graphic and/or offensive to some readers.

Acknowledgments

A s with any production, there are people to acknowledge who helped to accomplish the goal. Anyone who has been in the operating room or has seen office patients with me has heard me repeatedly say,

"An old surgeon once taught me…"

They weren't all old, but I must credit all the surgeons who spent their time trying to teach me even one tidbit of knowledge that I could use to help my patients.

I was converted in medical school from surgery to plastic surgery after spending time with John C. Kelleher, MD (Chief). I am truly indebted to him as he showed me the finesse of plastic surgery techniques in traumatic reconstructions and burns as well as aesthetic procedures. In each case, he pointed out the patient's happiness with the final improvements and how it affected their life. It was an experience early in my training to be able to witness firsthand the great effect plastic surgery has on the patient's life. The general surgeons in Boston taught me good surgical principles. The plastic surgeons in Baltimore drilled into me appropriate preoperative evaluations, intra-operative decision-making, and appropriate postoperative care. Most important, they also taught me how to manage patient expectations. Dr. A. Lee Dellon in particular started me on my academic career early by saying, "Just publish it, already."

I met Dr. Foad Nahai when I interviewed with him for a plastic surgery residency. My interview took place in the operating room as he corrected another plastic surgeon's complication. Little did I appreciate at that time that corrective surgery would be such a large part of my practice. The honesty and thoughtfulness of his presentations and writings helped me to develop my approach to plastic surgery procedures, and I have often stopped him to ask for his help with my more complex patients. Plastic surgeons from all over the world often tap into his knowledge and expertise. Dr. Nahai has a hard time maintaining good patient review ratings because he is frequently dragged from his patient office to help other plastic surgeons.

Dr. Joel Feldman was my mentor during my training in Boston. He allowed me to depart from my general surgery training responsibilities and taught me the precision and artistry needed to be a more thorough plastic surgeon, appreciating every nuance of patients and procedures.

I have to thank all the surgeons I have corralled at plastic surgery meetings for "just five minutes…I promise." These conversations often turn into 20-minute discussions over coffee. One conference that I attended yearly for 20 years was The Cutting Edge in New York City under the direction of Dr. Sherrell Aston and Dr. Daniel Baker. Many of the insights in this book are from Dr. Aston and Dr. Baker as well as from the numerous presenters and attendees. I humbly acknowledge all of their contributions.

To everyone I gave the preliminary manuscripts to read, I thank you for your opinions and insights. A shoutout to Mary Wamhoff, who put years of work into the manuscript, and Tiffany Guerra, who formatted the pictures and drawings. They have proved invaluable.

Also, thank you to my hardworking reviewer and editor, Lisbeth Tanz Goldberg, for tying it all together. She helped bring my manuscript out from under a pile of dust from neglect, and she changed the mumbo jumbo of a surgeon's writing into an easy-to-read book for everyone who may be contemplating having plastic surgery. Thanks, too, to Arlyn Lawrence and Chelsea Greenwood of Inspira Literary Solutions, who did the final proofing and manuscript formatting and helped take the manuscript across the finish line for submission to my publisher, Morgan James Publishing.

I owe many thanks to those who made the artistic contributions to the manuscript, including photographer Suzy Gorman, with whom I have worked for years; artist Terry Hinkle, who contributed the freehand drawings; Mary Lynn Brophy, who contributed the artwork for the book cover; and medical illustrator Vicki Freeman, who designed the anatomic drawings. Thank you for bringing to life the concepts I discuss in my book.

Foreword

I was pleased when Dr. Tom Francel, also known as "The Fixer," asked if I would write the foreword for this work. Having first met him when I was invited as a visiting professor to Johns Hopkins during his plastic surgery training, and since then witnessing his successful career, I readily accepted the task. Little did I know then that I would read the entire book before I could start clicking my keyboard. After all, skimming through the table of contents would have been enough to go on. The comprehensive table of contents whetted my appetite such that I started going through chapter after chapter. As I did so, I found myself nodding in agreement with every word and at the same time wanting everyone contemplating plastic surgery to also read every word. In particular, I wished that all those unfortunate victims of bad plastic surgery I have personally corrected over the years would have had access to such an informative resource before making that ill-advised choice the first time round.

To refer to this book as comprehensive is an understatement. Based on his extensive experience fixing bad plastic surgery, Dr. Francel has left nothing out. It would have sufficed had he covered the major reason why there is bad plastic surgery: the unqualified, underqualified, and inexperienced provider. He goes way beyond that in numerous chapters, discussing other contributing factors such as the media, real and or fake reviews, psychological issues, unrealistic expectations, and procedures that do not deliver. Beyond the clear and detailed explanations as to cause, he freely shares valuable advice and the secrets on how to avoid bad plastic surgery.

The writing is clear and readily comprehendible. The illustrations are well done and complement the words. I really enjoyed the quotes that are scattered over many of the pages.

I commend and thank Dr. Francel for undertaking this immense task, which will not only benefit the public and potential plastic surgery patients, but also our profession and especially our specialty. Bad plastic surgery reflects poorly on all of us plastic surgeons, as the public is not able to distinguish between those of us who are qualified and those who are not.

This work will go a long way in curtailing bad plastic surgery. It belongs in the hands of any woman or man contemplating plastic surgery and on the shelves of all practitioners.

Foad Nahai, MD, FACS, FRCS (hon)
Professor Plastic Surgery, Emory University, Atlanta, Georgia, USA; *Aesthetic Surgery Journal*, Editor in Chief (Emeritus); International Society of Aesthetic Plastic Surgery, past president; American Society for Aesthetic Plastic Surgery, past president; American Board of Plastic Surgery, former director; Plastic Surgery Research Council, past chairman; Author of over 200 peer-reviewed articles; editor or co-editor of eight textbooks in plastic surgery; editor and coauthor of the three-volume textbook *The Art of Plastic Surgery*

Introduction

Botched Up Bodies was initially broadcast in England in 2013 and highlighted bad plastic surgical results on patients the world over. Similarly, the *Botched* television series was a hit in in the US when it first aired on E! in the spring of 2014. The premise of the American series was that two surgeons, board-certified in their respective fields, were to evaluate and attempt to correct the results of botched or bad plastic surgery. Viewers of this series were fascinated by seeing these horrific results and listening to each patient's story to learn how they chose the outrageous procedures they requested and how they got botched.

But why did they get a botched result? Did these patients contribute to their problems, was it the procedure performed, or was it the result of who performed the procedure? "Yes" may be the answer to all of these questions.

If you choose to have plastic surgery, it's essential to understand why botched plastic surgery occurs and how to avoid a bad plastic surgery result. By reading this book, you should escape becoming an example patient on *Botched* or *Botched Up Bodies*.

One of the most significant issues contributing to bad plastic surgery is the large number of unqualified providers performing plastic surgery. A growing number of physicians without specialized training in plastic surgery are performing plastic surgery at the expense of results as well as patient safety. If you pay attention to the media and advertisements, it may seem like there are a plethora of plastic surgeons in US cities. However, at a recent plastic surgery meeting, researchers from New York University presented a study that visited websites resulting from the search "plastic surgeon." Of the sites visited, only 25 percent featured legitimate, board-certified plastic surgeons. In addition, over two thirds of recognized board-certified plastic surgeons didn't come up in the results. In fact, even I didn't show up!

This study concluded that a significant number of practitioners in the community are performing plastic surgery who aren't board-certified in plastic surgery. These people aren't plastic surgeons! In American print and electronic media, the majority of providers claiming to be plastic surgeons aren't qualified to make that claim. Their aim is to increase the number of patients coming to their offices for more lucrative plastic surgery procedures—even if that means they must mislead the public to achieve their goal.

These surgeons/physicians are misrepresenting themselves by inferring or directly stating that they have the training equivalent to a board-certified plastic surgeon. These providers typically list cosmetic surgery or aesthetic boards, which lack the vigorous training and testing required of board certification in plastic surgery. Their misrepresentation cheapens the title of "Plastic Surgeon." Now, it's possible that some of these potential providers are well trained. But it's much more likely that many are minimally trained or poorly trained to provide the service. While some providers look at you as a patient, others refer to you as a client.

Most consumers assume that all surgeons have the specialized training, credentials, and experience to perform plastic surgery procedures. Sadly, this may not be true. You have the right to know the qualifications of the provider you're entrusting your face, your body, as well as your life to—so ask them.

There's a turf war over who will provide your aesthetic procedures. You may be bombarded daily with advertisements from a variety of providers who want to improve your appearance and take your money. But is it really a turf war when it's a matter of safety? Shouldn't the educational requirements and training of the physician or the laypeople who perform even minor cosmetic procedures, chemical peels, and laser therapies, and inject fillers be clearly stated? Isn't your safety of the most importance?

It's my opinion that a board-certified physician should personally see and evaluate each patient, diagnose their problems, and establish the appropriate solutions before handing patient care to others. An increasing number of complications surrounding aesthetic procedures including burns, infections, tissue death, blindness, or even death have been occurring under the guise of plastic surgery. Is this because procedures are being administered improperly or done on an inappropriate patient? It seems really hard to object to increased oversight by a board-certified medical professional to lessen the risk to each patient.

I have over thirty years of experience as an established plastic surgeon, now practicing in St. Louis. I completed nine years of surgical training at Harvard Surgical Services in Boston and at Johns Hopkins Plastic Surgery Division in Baltimore before accepting a position as an attending surgeon at Washington University St. Louis, and Chief of Plastic Surgery at Jewish Hospital St. Louis. I have held academic appointments at Harvard Medical School, Johns Hopkins School of Medicine, Washington University School of Medicine St. Louis, and St. Louis University School of Medicine. I've been Chief of Plastic Surgery in all hospitals where I've worked and am presently in private practice at a level one trauma center in St. Louis, Missouri.

In 1993, after earlier obtaining board certification in General Surgery, I joined an elite group of plastic surgeons recognized by the American Board of Plastic Surgery. There have been fewer than 9,000 board-certified plastic surgeons in the United States since the board was first recognized in 1937. Presently, less than forty board-certified plastic surgeons are in active practice in the St. Louis metropolitan area, a region with a population of under three million people.

During my years as a plastic surgeon, I've seen a lot of bad plastic surgery, whether as a secondary consultant or on the streets of New York City, Los Angeles, Miami, Hong Kong, Sidney, London, Paris, Barcelona, and many other cities around the world. I used to shake my head as I walked by these odd-looking people, knowing that they didn't have to look that way. Plastic surgery, done in a measured way, improves appearances. When done with a heavy hand, odd-looking or sometimes inhuman-looking is the result. I knew I never wanted a patient of mine to look anything like these people. I thought I could help potential patients avoid bad results, and these ideas culminated in this book.

Today, approximately one third of my practice involves revision procedures from bad plastic surgery perpetrated by other physicians. My staff is often in the uncomfortable position of trying to distract a new facelift patient from staring at the botched facelift patient sitting across from them in the waiting room. A number of these first-time patients, in fact, have confessed to my staff that for a moment they were ready to run—not walk—out of the waiting room. One patient divulged that she never even entered the waiting room after looking in the waiting room window and seeing a bad result sitting there. She returned months later after the friend who referred her explained the situation, which was confirmed by a phone call to my staff.

Every patient has a story to tell about why they want to change their looks. Understanding their pain, frustration, fears, and hopes all figures into the education process I use as part of my initial and follow-up consultations with new patients. I believe it's my responsibility to educate them on what is and isn't possible, necessary, or even desirable to achieve their aesthetic goals. Most patients listen and understand. Others look for a surgeon to do their bidding regardless of the consequences.

What should be a plastic surgeon's ultimate goal for the patient? Contradictory advice includes:

- Plastic surgeons should make the patient look younger, not different.
- Plastic surgeons should be less concerned with making the patient look younger but make them look better.
- The best plastic surgery makes the patient look different but does not make the patient look strange or unrecognizable.

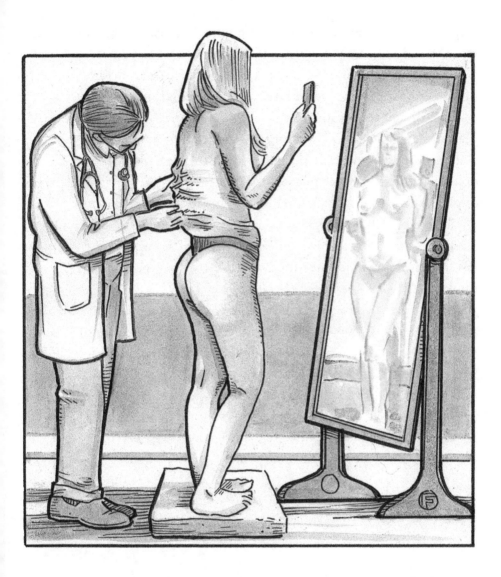

Patients come to me with different goals. Most want to look natural and not so different that people know they had plastic surgery the moment they walk into the room. But others have different goals. I had one patient whose daughter was graduating from graduate school, and she wanted to look as "young as possible." We performed surgery with that in mind, and she looked almost the same age as her daughter when we were done, but all of her present acquaintances absolutely knew that she had surgery done. At her next college reunion, all her classmates commented that she had not changed since graduation twenty years before.

But what is important is the patient's goal. The patient should decide his or her own personal goal and discuss this with the surgeon.

The thoughts and ideas in this book have been developed over my years of practicing as a plastic surgeon and from listening to both patients and surgeons. I've formulated many of these ideas through memorable experiences that I'll share with you. While all the ideas in this book aren't original, they all serve as cautionary and instructional information.

This book will help expose the causes of botched plastic surgery. It will teach you how to recognize and avoid bad plastic surgery and the poor results that follow poor decisions. You don't want people looking at you, thinking, *Oh no…Look what they had done!*

This book will offer guidance to help you obtain the best, most natural plastic surgery results possible. A good result will give you more self-confidence, an improved outward projection, and will cause others to say, "You look marvelous! Did you have something done?!"

Chapter 1

"Why Is There Sooo Much Bad Plastic Surgery"?

- - - - - - - - - - - -

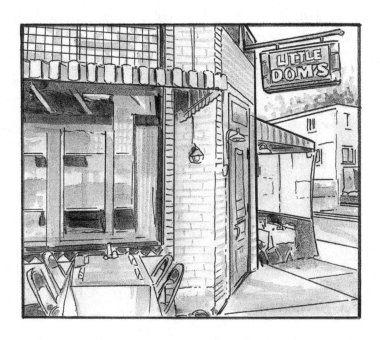

The idea to write this book originated from a conversation I had with Danielle, a Hollywood hairdresser and makeup consultant. We met at a private dinner party at Little Dom's restaurant in Los Angeles. When she discovered that I was a plastic surgeon, she asked me accusingly,

"Dude, why is there *sooo* much bad plastic surgery out there? Don't the people realize that it's bad? Don't they realize how bad they look?"

Although I'd thought about these questions over the years, Danielle's perspective was of particular interest to me. Like me, she deals with bad plastic surgery every day in her profession. Danielle walks onto Hollywood sets or into clients' homes and is stunned not only by unattractive surgical results but also by the results of too much Botox, fillers, and other less-invasive nonsurgical procedures. She uses her almost magical ability and expertise to camouflage the deformities she encounters to make her clients look normal and sometimes even pretty again.

You've seen some of Danielle's work on the red carpet as well as in the tabloids' "Stars with and without Makeup" photos. She asked me at dinner, "Some problems are impossible for me to correct, so why do surgeons do this to people?"

By the time dessert and coffee arrived, we'd both shared what we felt were reasons for "sooo much bad plastic surgery," and I knew that I needed to put these thoughts together to help others avoid bad plastic surgery.

After meeting Danielle, I started collecting information on botched plastic surgery, analyzing why it happens, and strategizing as to how patients can avoid it.

A Brief Description of Plastic Surgery

Many people are confused about the terms "plastic surgery," "cosmetic surgery," and "aesthetic surgery." Cosmetic and aesthetic surgery may be used interchangeably and both may be considered part of plastic surgery. Aesthetic surgery deals with appearances and focuses on beauty. It's considered a specialty within plastic surgery. Plastic surgery includes both aesthetic surgery and reconstructive surgery. Aesthetic surgery improves upon the appearance of normal structures whereas reconstructive surgery attempts to reconstruct or restore congenital, traumatic, or disease-altered structures back to a normal appearance or to normal functioning structures.

Decades ago, there were fewer plastic surgeons and they were generally well trained. They learned their artistic and technical skills through reconstructive procedures designed to bring abnormal structures back to normalcy. They had an excellent concept of the difference between normal and abnormal. Older surgeons taught me most of these historical procedures, and I've used them for years. I learned many of the newer procedures from presentations at plastic surgery conferences and perfected them in the anatomy lab before performing them on my patients.

Origins of Bad Plastic Surgery

Presently, some providers of plastic surgery have lost the ability or the desire to differentiate between good plastic surgery, which reestablishes aesthetic features, and bad plastic surgery. Bob Beckel, a TV and radio commentator, once commented about walking into a Florida restaurant with so many examples of bad plastic surgery that it was like "walking into a room from *Night of the Living Dead.*" It's as though people have become so used to seeing bad plastic surgery that they expect it, not realizing a more natural improvement can be the result from plastic surgery done well.

Bad plastic surgery results from three influences: the patient, the provider, and the procedure chosen. The patient may try to dictate the procedure performed, and some patients want to look *done* or *different*. Poorly trained providers perform a lot of the bad plastic surgery you may encounter. What keeps these people in business are the patients who keep coming to them often because of the lower costs charged for procedures. This book examines each of these influences, analyzes why each happens, and discusses what the patient can do to prevent an unfavorable result.

But Be Safe!

Patients need to embrace the positive aesthetic improvements and improved quality of life that good plastic surgery delivers. But patients must also consider their safety during their quest for improvement. In 2014, the plastic surgery industry lost Joan Rivers, a great ambassador for the merits of plastic surgery. She died because the clinic where she was undergoing a procedure to evaluate voice changes and stomach reflux didn't have the necessary lifesaving equipment and drugs normally present during surgery. When the comedian suffered cardiac arrest, the facility's staff didn't act quickly enough to prevent her unnecessary death. The cautionary tale here is to fully evaluate the facility, physician, and procedures in place for surgery and emergencies before moving ahead with an aesthetic improvement.

As a comparison, a prominent St. Louis figure was undergoing a procedure at our hospital's surgery center similar to what Joan Rivers had done. An instrument was passed into the patient's lungs and stomach to evaluate his heartburn symptoms and frequent pneumonia. It was thought that his stomach contents were regurgitating (aspirating) into his lungs. His airway swelled, which stopped the airflow into his lungs. A surgeon operating two rooms over was called in to surgically establish an emergency airway (cricothyrotomy), thereby saving the patient's life.

If you take one thing from this book, I hope it's how to remain safe. I've lost count of how many patients I've treated who were admitted into our emergency room with life-threatening complications following aesthetic procedures performed in freestanding surgery centers and physicians' offices. An emergency room visit wasn't what these patients were expecting, but it happens more often than you'd think.

On one occasion, a patient arrived in distress from a doctor's office after a neck liposuction procedure. The patient was bleeding into his neck, which was compromising his airway. He required an immediate emergency airway, which we performed in our emergency room. Turns out, the physician who performed the procedure had no hospital or operating room privileges at any facility. Worse, this provider wasn't even a surgeon! Yet, his advertisements claimed he had board certification in cosmetic surgery. This patient had to be transported via ambulance to our high-level care emergency room for a lifesaving procedure because his physician couldn't save him.

In another example, I treated a woman who arrived by ambulance from her gynecologist's office. The gynecologist had perforated the patient's abdominal wall at least ten times during a liposuction procedure. The patient came in with peritonitis, a life-threatening condition that required one surgery to save her life and two more to reconnect her injured bowel.

Another patient arrived after a tummy tuck done at a surgery center with an abdominal wall so full of blood that she had little blood left in her circulatory system to support the rest of her body. Her blood pressure had fallen low enough to threaten her life. She was saved only by an emergency resuscitation by our in-hospital anesthesiologist and an urgent operation.

An ear, nose, and throat doctor sent a severely ill patient to our emergency with a freshly placed breast implant on the right side. On the left, the patient had a collapsed lung. The emergency occurred after an attempted breast augmentation by an unqualified surgeon.

No one undergoes plastic surgery expecting to end up in the emergency room. Your safety must be your main concern as you consider procedures and the physicians who may perform them. In fact, each time I see a complication like this, I am reminded of a warning an attending surgeon said to me during my general surgery training: "Never perform any procedure for which you would be incapable of treating any and all of the potential complications."

Still Look Like You

For many people, the word "plastic" means artificial, fake, phony, or put-on. The misconception is that a "plastic surgery" procedure transforms that person's natural appearance into something artificial, synthetic, fake, or unnatural. Even my dear mother thought aesthetic surgery patients looked "plastic or fake." But "plastic surgery" should remodel or refine a patient's outward appearance and doesn't need to look artificial, fake, or even weird.

This book will help you navigate the world of plastic surgery, and its contents are designed to educate readers on how to avoid bad plastic surgery. You don't want to be the person people notice because you've obviously had work done.

A fellow plastic surgeon once told me she encountered such a person at her high school reunion. Upon meeting her former classmate, my colleague frantically looked at the woman's high school picture and the name on her badge to help identify her. Her classmate looked nothing like her senior picture. All her distinguishable features from back then were gone from her face. It was obvious she'd had extensive plastic/rejuvenation surgery. Although she had been one of the prettier classmates in high school, now she looked tight, puffy, and distorted. She'd lost her original uniqueness with stereotypical bad plastic surgery performed on her eyes, nose, and face. Her breasts were also too big, too high, and too close together for her age. She was the talk of the reunion but not in a flattering way. Most of the other attendees commented, "I don't think she looks better, but she sure looks different."

Don't let that person be you! People should notice you because you're attractive with no clue that you've had a little help getting there. Or you might prefer that they say, "You look fabulous! Who did it, and how much was it?"

Chapter 2
The Public Perception of Plastic Surgery

- - - - - - - - - - -

Comedians Joan Rivers and Phyllis Diller were both famous for making fun of themselves and their many plastic surgeries. Their comedy highlighted the love/hate relationship people seem to have with having "work done" on the face and body. A few years ago, I had an encounter that illustrates the negative perception the public has about plastic surgery and plastic surgeons. Ironically, it also shows how good plastic surgery can really be.

On this evening, I had a dinner date with friends at a local steak house. I arrived early, and since it was cold outside, I decided to go in and grab a glass of wine at the bar. Inside, a couple was sitting on a bench waiting for a table. I recognized the woman as an operating room nurse at my hospital. She also happened to be my patient. Ordinarily, I won't approach one of my patients in a public venue unless they initially talk to me. I want to maintain their privacy so there's no need to explain to their friends why they know the plastic surgeon. However, I knew her professionally, so I felt safe approaching her and saying, "Hi." Our conversation started out pleasant enough.

"Hi, Sarah. I'm Tom Francel." As I said this, I reached out to shake her husband's hand. Sarah smiled and said hello. After that, it was all her husband.

"It seems my wife knows a lot of younger men. How do you know her?"

"I'm a plastic surgeon and work with her in the operating room," I replied.

"A what?!" he exclaimed. "So, you're one of those plastic surgeons who change people and make them look weird." His tone was accusatory.

"Well, we actually try to make them look better," I said with a smile.

"Better? Hah! They all look weird. God didn't make people so you could change them. As a physician, you should be saving lives, not this crap that you do." He seemed very pleased with himself.

I quickly flashed back to my general surgery training and recalled suturing a stab wound to the heart of an 18-year-old boy, saving his life. In my plastic surgery training, I'd reattached ears, arms, fingers, legs, and even penises. I kept those memories to myself.

"In my surgery training, I've saved many lives. But now I perform reconstructive and cosmetic surgery procedures, all of which are meant to improve the quality of people's lives. These patients behave more confidently, engage more often, and appear happier. I now help people be happy about themselves."

He responded, "What a bunch of baloney!"

Seeing this was only going in the wrong direction, I ended our conversation by shaking his hand. I think that caught him off guard, as he returned the pleasantry. During this exchange, Sarah looked embarrassed. She didn't look up, but instead stared at the floor. She was a long-term aesthetic patient of mine, having undergone multiple office procedures. After my exchange with her husband, I was sure she'd never told him about any them. By his comments, it was obvious he didn't know she'd had anything done. She was pretty, and probably did attract a lot of younger men, yet because there weren't any unnatural distortions, he was totally clueless that she'd undergone any aesthetic procedures. That is the way it can and should be.

Since I'm a board-certified plastic surgeon, I see reconstruction patients in my office (breast reconstruction after cancer, face reconstruction after oral or skin cancer, chest reconstruction after cancer or infection, etc.) as well as aesthetic patients. Some of these reconstruction patients even question me as to why I perform these "crazy" cosmetic surgeries when I devote so much of my time to reconstruction patients. These anti-aesthetic surgery patients say,

- "I want to show my emotions."
- "People should have their natural nose and not those fake-looking noses."
- "I've worked hard for every line and wrinkle."
- "People at sixty shouldn't look like they're forty or even fifty years old."
- "Aging is part of life, and you should look your age."

Even my dear mother joined into that line of questioning and asked me why I do this "looking-good" surgery.

Plastic Surgery Shouldn't Scream; It Should Whisper

The goal of having plastic surgery is to create a positive change in a person's appearance and life. It can make people feel and look better and doesn't have to look "plastic" or unnatural. Good plastic surgery should produce appropriate changes and improvements. The plastic surgery patient should still be recognized at school reunions yet appear refreshed and look vibrant, energetic, and as though time has stood still.

The public perception, as exhibited by Sarah's husband, is strongly suggested by the media and doesn't reveal the broad scope of plastic surgery as a surgical subspecialty. In essence, plastic surgery is restorative. It corrects the effects of aging (aesthetics) but it also restores and corrects structures that were deformed either congenitally at birth or due to cancer, accidents, and infections. It also restores a patient's love of life, vigor, and self-confidence.

Most people will correctly identify plastic surgeons as performing tummy tucks, facelifts, eyelid surgery, nasal surgeries, breast augmentation, and liposuction. It's less understood by the public that plastic surgeons also perform breast reconstructions, burn reconstruction, cleft lip and palate repairs, facial and skull deformity corrections in children, wound repairs and closures, and hand surgery including bone injuries.

Plastic surgery is limited only by the borders of the human body. Plastic surgeons work in the head and neck, the extremities, and the trunk. Because of our extensive training, we can reconstruct:

- The skull and the scalp;
- The face including, transplantation;
- The arms and legs, including replantation of lost limbs or parts;
- The chest, including reconstruction after breast cancer as well as infections around the heart and lungs or the spine;
- The abdominal wall, as well as harvest intra-abdominal structures (bowel or omentum) to use as functional organs elsewhere; and
- Penises, vaginas, and pelvic floors by moving muscle and skin.

In fact, the first kidney transplantation was conceptualized and performed by a plastic surgeon in Boston in 1954 between identical twins. Dr. Joe Murray went on to perform the first successful cadaver kidney transplant in 1962. In 1990, he received the Nobel Prize in Medicine for his work in transplantation.

The plastic surgeon must have knowledge of disease in every part of the human body because plastic surgeons are the ones who are called on to reconstruct all body structures. Plastic surgeons are the last physician you'll see to help you return to normalcy after disease or injury, whether that's for function or physical appearance.

Sarah has witnessed the power of plastic surgery to repair and transform. She's helped me in the operating room in the wee hours of the morning reconstructing a face blown apart by a gunshot. She's passed implants to me for breast reconstruction after mastectomies for breast cancer. She's assisted in reconstructing the face of a homeless clinic patient whose cheekbone was removed for an ignored aggressive skin cancer. She's gotten me a cup of water to sip while I was under the microscope putting fingers back on the hand of a retired carpenter after a table-saw accident. Sarah has helped me perform a secondary cleft nasal reconstruction on an infant born with a cleft lip and palette. She's helped prepare a skin graft with me to cover a foot crushed by a forklift. But she's also assisted on many cosmetic procedures including facelifts, breast augmentations, and tummy tucks.

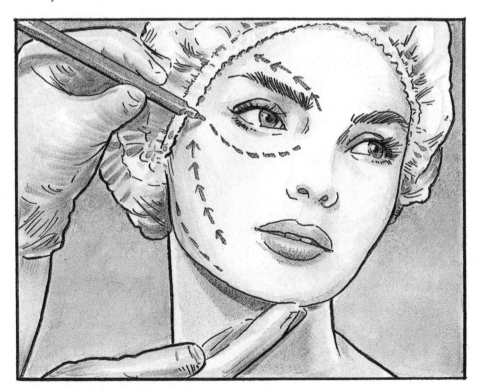

Such is plastic surgery. It is surgery of aesthetics as well as the reconstruction of deformed and injured parts of the body. It encompasses all ages, all genders, and all body areas. A good result is frequently uplifting to the patient's spirit. It adds to their happiness regardless whether the surgery is performed for cosmetic reasons or for reconstructive purposes. A postoperative patient behaves more confidently, is less introverted, and appears happier to everyone.

It was pretty obvious from my conversation that Sarah's husband also didn't know that his daughter Emily had undergone a breast augmentation, liposuction, and a tummy tuck done by me three years earlier. The fact that he didn't know this makes that good plastic surgery to me.

Good results are something we all strive for. So, "Why is there sooo much bad plastic surgery?"

Chapter 3
Natural and Aesthetic Ideals

The object of the artist is the creation of the beautiful. What the beautiful is is another question.

–James Joyce

We should be trying to avoid bad plastic surgery, but what is it exactly? Similar to pornography, you know it when you see it, but it's hard to describe. The attendees at the aforementioned high school reunion *knew* that their classmate didn't look like herself and looked *bad*. Why did they recognize her plastic surgery results as bad while she must have felt that she looked good? She may have even had the surgery in preparation for this big event. Why do some people recognize and avoid bad plastic surgery and yet others succumb to it?

Instead of attempting to define bad plastic surgery, let's define what constitutes good plastic surgery. By giving you a foundational understanding of what good plastic surgery is and how it's accomplished, you'll be in a much better position to avoid bad plastic surgery.

Good plastic surgery attempts to reverse the impact of aging and to restore features to create a more youthful appearance. This applies to the face and neck, breasts, abdominal wall, and extremities. As plastic surgeons, we should enhance each patient's features and assets to show beauty without radically altering the patient's appearance.

We can attempt to define aesthetically pleasing features mathematically by appreciating the body's inherent qualities. A good plastic surgeon respects proportions and aesthetic ratios and seeks to maintain each tissue's individual characteristic to maintain the body's gentle and soft quality. When the aesthetic numerical ratios or the softness of the tissues are interfered with, a surgeon may make the patient more artificial and even less pretty.

How Is a Beautiful Face Defined?

People realize when another person is beautiful, but it is difficult to adequately define *why* there's beauty. In the female face, some features are considered attractive: large eyes, greater distance between the eyes, high cheekbones with full cheeks, petite nose, decreased mouth width, full lips, and a smaller chin. In the male face, attractive features include a tall, prominent forehead, heavy brows and full upper eyelids, strong cheekbones with cheek hollows, substantial nose, oval-shaped face, angled jawline, and a full chin.

Beauty isn't only in the eye of the beholder, but also in the relationships between facial structures. The important proportions between facial features include between the forehead, eyes, nose, mouth, chin, and ears. A person's beauty may increase if their facial features are considered aesthetically proportional. We don't inherently know why there's beauty in these relationships, but it may be the result of people averaging the ratios of the many faces seen throughout childhood and beyond. Over the years, people then develop an appreciation of the *ideal ratios* seen in beautiful people. But can beauty be mathematical if each person's perception of beauty is different? The Greeks first used these beautiful aesthetic mathematical ratios, which they called *phi*, in their art, statues, and architecture. In the Middle Ages and Renaissance, a *divine proportion* was adopted, which was confirmed in the human body as ratios between bones, muscles, and many body structures.

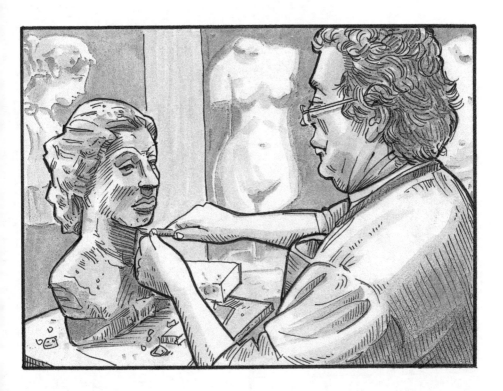

The divine aesthetic ratio is 1.62, which is found by measuring the distance between the various facial features. Dividing the length of the face (hairline to chin) by the width (ear to ear) should result in the golden ratio of 1.62, meaning, the length should be 1.62 to the width of 1. This ratio is also seen when measuring the eye to the teeth and the teeth to the chin. It is also evident when measuring the width of the eye to the distance from the inner eye to the center of the nose. Try these measurements on yourself to see how you fit into the aesthetic golden ratio of 1.62.

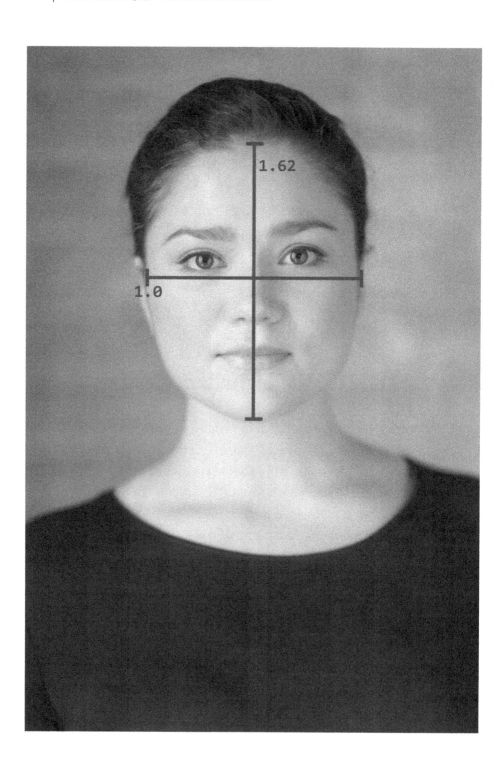

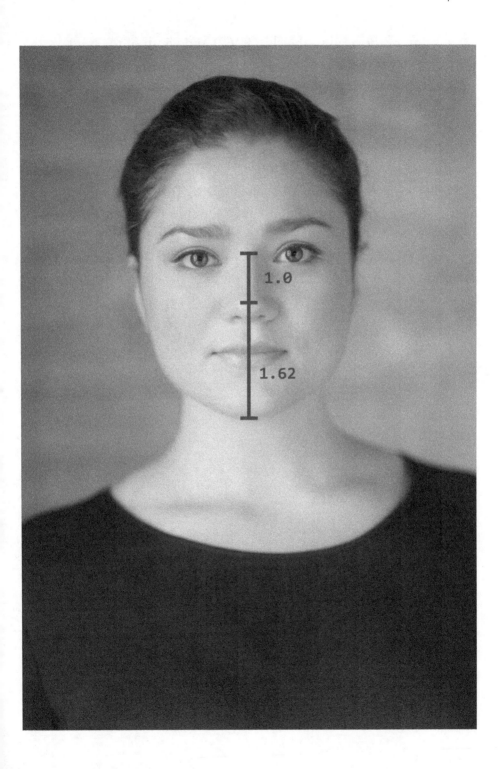

- Top of the head to the chin (1.62) and width of the head from ear to ear (1.0)
- Top of the head to the pupil and the pupil to the lip
- Nose tip to chin and lip separation to the chin
- Nose tip to the chin and pupil to nose tip
- Vertical height of the lower lip to the upper lip

There are also aesthetic ratios equaling 1.0. The length of the forehead hairline to the center of the pupils and the pupils to the base of the nose, and the base of the nose to the chin should all be in a 1.0 ratio, meaning, these three sections should all measure equally. The length of the ear equals the length of the nose, and the width of the eye equals the distance between the eyes.

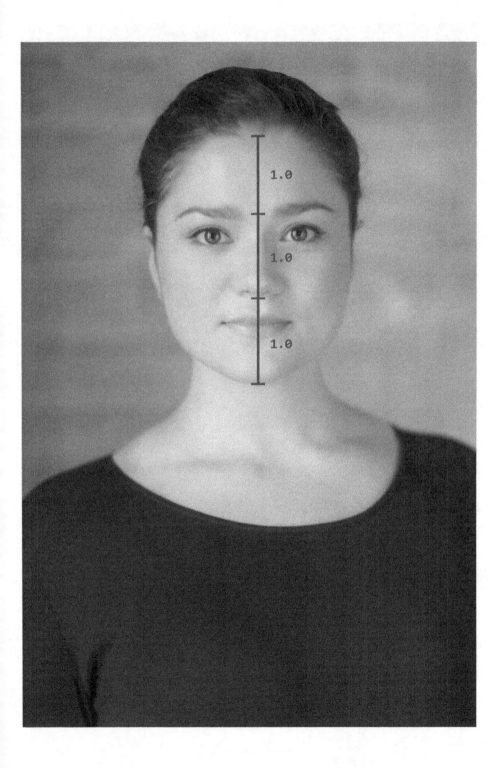

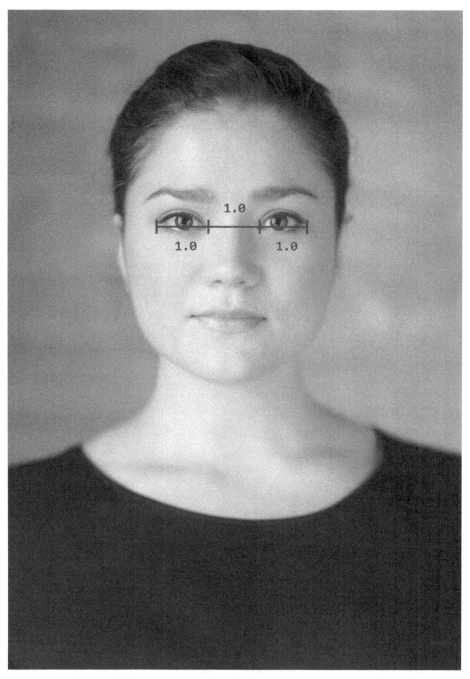

Some vertical relationships also exist in an aesthetically pleasing face, and these points should line up on the vertical.

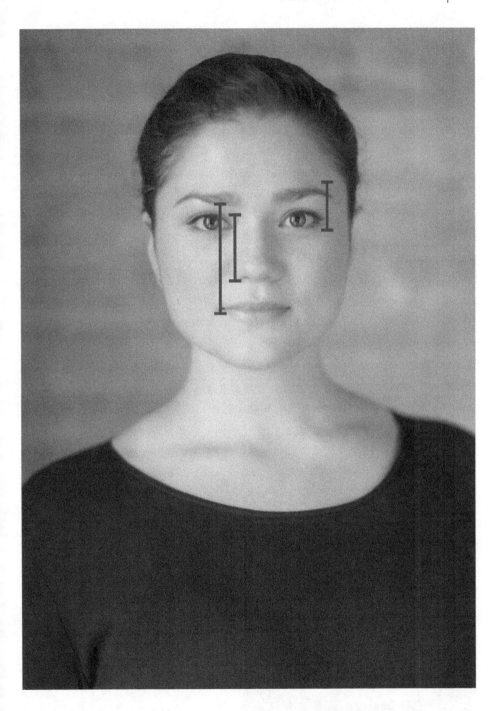

These include:

- The line between the base of the nose and the inner eye and the inside of the eyebrow
- The line between the outer eye and the eyebrow peak
- The line between the pupils and the outer corner of the mouth
- The width of the nose and the distance between the eyes

A more complex mathematical analysis was developed in 1997 by plastic surgeon Stephen Marquardt.[1] The Marquardt Beauty Analysis is a product of the Marquardt Foundation, which is a non-profit organization that provides treatment plans to physicians treating patients with facial aesthetic problems. Dr. Marquardt developed the Marquardt Beauty Mask believing that beauty is the combination of the golden ratio proportions in many facial markers as well as symmetry. In his analysis, the most important markers are the positions of the eyes, nose, mouth, chin, and eyebrows. It's amazing to see how the Marquardt Beauty Mask, when placed on attractive females, aligns perfectly with their features.

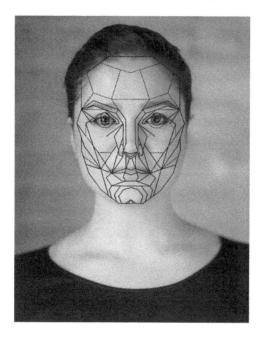

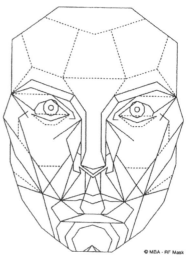

© MBA - RF Mask

Based on these analyses, small differences can dramatically alter a person's attractiveness. If one or two structures don't have the correct ratio or don't fit a golden triangle, then the person may not appear very pretty. But strategic millimeter corrections of the facial structures may make the person attractive or cute without radically altering their appearance. However, millimeter differences done without consideration of the person's overall appearance, especially in nasal surgery and eyelid surgery, can result in bad plastic surgery.

Symmetry isn't always necessary for when defining beauty. In fact, a slight asymmetry may be more beautiful than absolute symmetry because most people are somewhat asymmetric in their facial features, breasts, and other body regions. Acceptance of asymmetry is more a function of what we're used to seeing and appreciating. Extreme asymmetries, however, may be seen as unattractive. In other words, we may not expect perfection in others' appearance, but they should come pretty darn close.

Besides mathematically attractive features, other features represent youthfulness. These include bigger lips, bigger eyes, wider-set eyes, full eyebrows, and soft, round cheeks. These indicators reflect the appeal of a baby's round face with big eyes, small nose and chin, and soft round features—things that make us all smile.

Disrupting the Standards of Beauty

A face, like a signature, is unique. It has a recognizable look and is our distinct proof of identity. Good facial rejuvenation surgery will create small changes and restore an improved version of the self. Bad facial plastic surgery radically alters a person's appearance, making that person unrecognizable like the classmate at her high school reunion.

The loose skin of a stereotypical bad facelift patient has been pulled tightly in inappropriate vectors, which ignores the aging of the deeper fat and muscles. This is the post-facelift patient whose skin is pulled so tight that it looks like they've put their face outside a car window going 60 miles per hour. The forehead lift patient may look perpetually surprised. Poorly done eyelid surgery may leave the patient looking distrustful with beady eyes. Without concern for proportions, a patient may have a nose that looks too small or short and upturned for their facial structure and features. The Daily Mail Reporter in 2009 reported some nicknames for results of bad facial plastic surgery.[2] They include:

- Ping pong face—lumps from injectable material
- Bat brow—extreme arched eyebrows
- Wind tunnel—skin pulled too tight
- Trout pout—overinflated lips
- Horse mouth—overfilled perioral area
- Pillow face—overinflation of the cheeks with fillers

These are all avoidable problems.

A performance artist in France, who wants to disrupt the standards of beauty, is defying the importance of ratios and balance over individual parts. Using her body as her canvas, ORLAN has used body modification (plastic surgery) not to appear better, but to distort her appearance so that she appears different. She is not against plastic surgery, but rather against its conventions. She has transformed herself by recreating herself through alienation. Since 1990, she's used seven plastic surgeries to obtain her goal. Using beautiful female prototypes from classical works of art, ORLAN has transformed her appearance. Her face now displays the classic Greek nose from the statues of the huntress Diana, the mouth of Boucher's Europa, the forehead highlights of da Vinci's Mona Lisa, the chin from Botticelli's Rising Venus, and the eyes from Gerome's Psyche. Individually, these are all classic beauty parts. Put together, they lose their attractiveness.

ORLAN's facial modifications show that beauty isn't necessarily the sum of the parts, but rather how the parts relate to each other and maintain aesthetic ratios and relationships. Facial attractiveness is a balance of facial features not just the existence of attractive parts.

How Are Beautiful Breasts Defined?

The beautiful breast is defined by gentle, soft contours and flowing curves. These characteristics need to be maintained with plastic surgery. There is a subtle fullness and roundness reflecting back to the beauty of a round, full baby's face. Each breast should be a fully rounded, hemispheric structure on the chest wall with volume and contour in harmony with the trunk and buttock proportions. Two thirds of the breast tissue should be below the nipple with the greatest point of projection at the nipple. The areola (pigmented area containing the nipple) should be small and not stretched, which occurs with pregnancy. The fold below the breast should define the lowest point of breast tissue on the chest wall.

While slight asymmetry is acceptable in the face, it's not acceptable in the breasts. That's because asymmetry reduces the attractiveness of the chest area and may make the breasts appear older. To determine the aesthetic symmetry of breasts, a bit of geometry is employed.

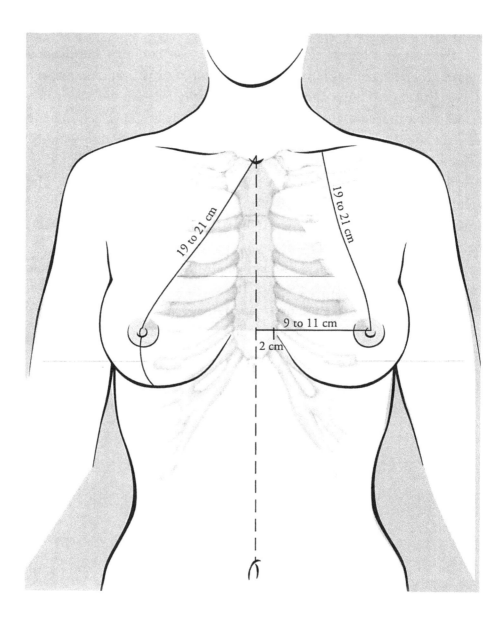

The generally accepted measurement for the attractive chest is a perfect isosceles triangle of 20 centimeters (roughly eight inches) from the base of the neck to each nipple and between each nipple. The breast typically starts about one inch from the midline, giving an approximate two-inch separation between the breasts over the breastbone. Therefore, cleavage doesn't exist naturally and needs to be made by artificially pushing the breasts upward and toward the midline. The nipple is about four to five inches from the midline. The diameter of the breast averages approximately four to six inches.

As the breasts age, they settle downward and toward the outside edge of the body. Their shape is now influenced by the woman's skin quality and her breast volume. As our skin ages, it becomes less elastic and prone to drooping and the development of stretch marks. The breast gland itself settles downward, flattening the upper part of the breast, which leads to a hollowing of the upper breast segment. As the breast tissue continues to descend, it obscures the lower breast fold when viewed from the front.

Good plastic surgery recreates the natural appearance and soft contours of the breast. It maintains body proportion, establishes symmetry, and keeps the scars hidden. The surgeon needs to understand each individual's anatomy and work through these differences to attain the ideal breast. This applies to breast augmentation as well as lifts, reductions, and reconstruction after surgical elimination of the breast for cancer treatment.

On the other hand, bad plastic surgery of the breasts results in unusual breast contours, extreme projection, and excessive upper fullness. Some patients ask for the *bouncing beach ball* breasts on some pornography stars. To achieve this extreme cleavage, the surgeon must place the implants near the midline of the chest. Doing so can cause the implants to be pushed so close together that a natural separation between the breasts is eliminated, creating a *uniboob* (one boob). Placing breasts in this way means they now extend beyond the existing natural breast contour. Others project out too much for their base footprint or rest high above the nipple (remember, only one third should be above the nipple), creating excessive and unnatural upper-breast fullness.

What Is an Attractive Abdominal Wall?

The contemporary standard of abdominal wall beauty is a muscular, toned, slender appearance with well-defined bony boundaries of the ribs and pelvic bones. This is contrary to the 14th and 15th centuries when plump, full, and overflowing abdomens were in fashion. Today's standard is more in line with the muscular abdominal wall of classical Greek and Roman statues. The present aesthetic abdominal wall is also a far cry from the skinny abdominal wall which was prevalent and desirable in the 1960s or the corseted abdomens of the 16th and 17th centuries.

The abdomen consists of the iliac crest, which is the area between the ribs and pelvis, and the midline, the larger area between the chest and pubis. The umbilicus (belly button) is on the midline at the level of the iliac crest and has an overlying hood of skin. The waist, just above the umbilicus, is the narrowest part of the abdomen. The midline overall is a depressed hollow midline with muscle definition ending at the mons pubis, which is elevated over the central pelvic bones.

People are either short or long waisted.

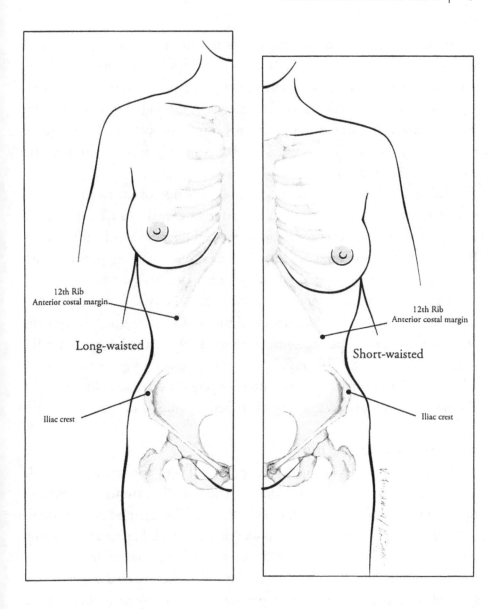

The terms "short waisted" or "long waisted" come from the measurable distance between the lower rib cage to the iliac crest. A short waist means only five to six centimeters separate those two areas. In a long waist, the distance between them is closer to ten or eleven centimeters. It's difficult to create an ideal abdominal wall if the person is short waisted. Some surgeons try to convert a short waist to a long waist by removing the lower ribs.

Improvements in the abdominal wall with a tummy tuck are best accomplished when the skin is flaccid, the muscles are strong, and there's a paucity of soft tissue. The best patients are postpartum with muscle separation, a lower abdominal skin excess, and good skin tone without stretch marks. Attempted improvements using liposuction alone requires elastic skin and muscle definition, which is usually seen in women who haven't carried children.

Bad abdominal surgery occurs when liposuction of the fat under loose skin is attempted, but the person has poorly defined muscles. The result is a "turkey tummy" where the stomach resembles a flaccid turkey neck. Because of the contemporary standard of beauty, heavier patients with unrealistic expectations are requesting tummy tucks. For these patients, a positive outcome is difficult to achieve because often, the abdominal fat surrounding the internal organs limits the results, even though the fat directly underneath the skin is removed. Some of the most horrific results occur when a post-tummy tuck patient gains a significant amount of weight (50 pounds or more) after surgery. The fat remaining in the abdominal cavity grows, creating unattractive lumps and bumps.

How Are Hips Beautiful?

Waist and hip measurements are seen as a major contributor to female attractiveness. The waist measurement is taken at the narrowest segment of the waist just above the umbilicus (belly button). The tightness of the abdominal muscles and the amount of fat under the skin will influence this measurement. Tight muscles and less fat will decrease the waist measurement.

The hip measurement is taken at the widest section of the pelvis, typically at the hip and pubis level. Contributing anatomy includes the bone structures (pelvis and hip bones) and the soft tissue (muscles and fat). The more open the pelvis, the stronger and larger the buttock muscles, and the more fat that's present, the higher the hip measurement. It's been determined that a waist-to-hip ratio (WHR) of 0.70 plays an important role in the initial attraction of a male to a female.

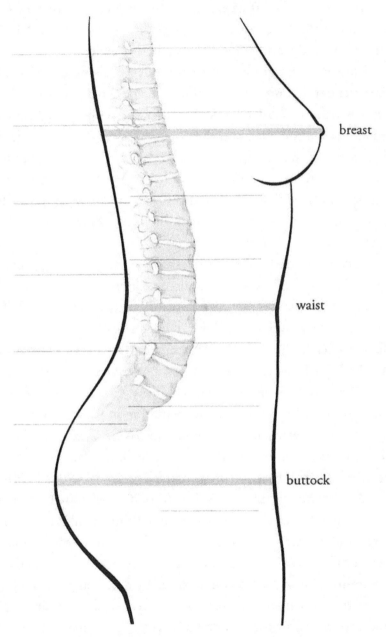

breast

waist

buttock

The aesthetic ratio of the torso includes the waist-to-hips ratio (WHR) of 0.70. The breast-to-hips ratio should be 1.0.

This ratio of 0.70 approaches the aesthetic ratio 0.62 (or 1.62) as seen in beautiful facial features. Quite differently, a male WHR of 0.90 is important in the attraction of a female to a male.

Most men prefer slender, curvaceous female figures with a low WHR over slender figures with a tubular shape (high WHR). It is felt that females with a WHR of 0.70, whether the female was heavy or slender, are more feminine than figures with a lower WHR and a larger breast size. This suggests that an appropriate WHR of 0.70 is more important and more attractive to men than even a long-legged, small-hipped, and busty Barbie-doll type. Consider the measurements of 36-24-36. A bust size of 36 is a one-to-one proportion with the hips, which is ideal. The WHR is at the magic number of 0.70.

You don't need to have the above measurements to be considered attractive. The WHR works well for different-sized bodies. Successful, established models over the years consistently show a 0.70 WHR despite changes in body weight. The overall body size of attractive models through the last decades has decreased (compare Marilyn Monroe to Kate Moss), yet the WHR has remained remarkably consistent at 0.70. Because the WHR is a comparison between two measurements, two women can have the same WHR in spite of a wide variation in waist or hip size. A woman with a thicker waist and large hips can have a WHR of 0.70 similar to a woman with a narrow waist and smaller hips. Many recent models are described as "full sized" yet have attractive curves with a WHR of 0.70.

Besides attractiveness, a WHR of 0.70 is also linked to better health and thereby perceived increased fertility. Prior to puberty, a female's WHR is very tubular and man-like at 0.90. After puberty, sex hormones distribute fat differently in each sex. Female estrogen concentrates fat around the hips, pubis, buttocks, and thighs, thereby decreasing the WHR to around 0.70. In comparison, testosterone increases fat deposition around the midsection and in the abdominal cavity (i.e., core fat) and increases the WHR. A proper WHR suggests that a woman is in better health because she's able to appropriately store fat. Therefore, she's more fertile with a greater chance of successful childbirth because she has "good childbearing hips" and a more open pelvis. Compare this to a non-menstruating female marathon runner with a tubular body.

But as females age beyond menopause, fat is lost in the buttocks and thighs. The previously full skin becomes lax and drooping. The firm and round youthful buttock changes to a lax, flat, and square buttock with a high WHR. In an attempt to reverse aging, more women are amending their ratio by increasing their hip measurement with the help of implants or fat grafting. This may also be performed for aesthetic considerations when a patient's waist measurement may be too large to obtain a more attractive ratio. In fact, buttock augmentation is one of the fastest growing aesthetic procedures.

Chapter 4

Recent Increases in Plastic Surgery Procedures

- - - - - - - - - - - -

There's an old saying "you can never be too rich or too thin." Now the feeling seems to be that "you can never be too inflated, too smooth, too tight, or too buxom." Most people are unhappy with at least one part of their body, and many would pursue surgery to change what concerns them. The number of total cosmetic surgical procedures decreased by 14 percent during the Covid pandemic. Breast augmentation dropped the most during this period (about 30 percent). Minimally invasive cosmetic procedures (neuromodulators, fillers, lasers, etc.) also decreased about 17 percent. But the total projected numbers for 2022 appear to be returning to pre-Covid total numbers

Plastic surgery procedures have increased over the last few years. As reported by the American Society of Plastic Surgeons, Americans had over 17.7 million cosmetic procedures (up 2 percent from 2017) at a total expenditure of about eighteen billion dollars (up 20 percent) in 2018.[3] This is a sixfold increase since 1997. These numbers are only the procedures reported by board-certified plastic surgeons and don't include other providers. Perhaps not surprisingly, those between the ages of forty and fifty-five account for 49 percent of procedures, followed by those over fifty-five at 25 percent, and, finally, those twenty to thirty-nine years old at 22 percent. About 92 percent of the procedures are performed on females.

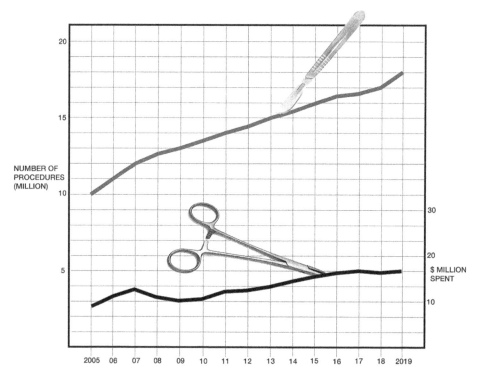

The graphs show progressive increase as well as money spent
for plastic surgery procedures.

The Driving Force

So, what's driving the recent increase in people undergoing plastic/ cosmetic surgery? One reason is the increase in coverage of plastic surgery by the media. Examples of the latest and greatest cosmetic procedures are favorite topics in style, health, and beauty magazines as well as daytime chat shows. The Kardashian/Jenner family, in their show *Keeping Up with the Kardashians*, exposed the public to skin care, facial fillers, Botox, cosmetic office procedures, and plastic surgery. The present-day media is hyping all these "advances" in plastic surgery, and it seems like everyone is doing it.

The discussion has even advanced from *rejuvenation* to *prejuvenation*—the attempt to prevent aging by starting interventions at an early age.

Surgically altered faces are ubiquitous in our present multimedia culture and are much more accepted than they were ten years ago. Just look at newscasters, soap stars, TV hosts, and reality show stars. Today, people realize that youthful beauty is something that can be bought and enjoyed, an understanding that's reinforced by commercials for popular cosmetic products and procedures that wouldn't have been aired that many years ago. In the past, women were less likely to reveal that they'd had surgery, let alone allow their pictures to be used in commercials, on TV, and in magazines.

Society places a great deal of pressure on women to look younger and sexier. Yet, society has labeled women as superficial for caring too much about their appearance or selfish for indulging themselves with expensive plastic surgery, too. As the approval of plastic surgery has increased, the stigma of "going under the knife" has decreased, making it more acceptable for women to alter their appearance.

Women are now more aware of what cosmetic surgery may do for a women's psyche. Patients reveal this by statements such as:

- I'm finally doing something for myself.
- I'm gaining confidence.
- I'm improving myself.
- I feel better about myself.
- I care *about* myself so I care *for* myself.

Studies have shown that the benefits of plastic surgery go beyond just physical appearance and include improvements in body image and self-esteem.[4] Almost 90 percent of patients continue to be happy with their improvements even one year after surgery. The patients also reported a significant improvement in body image especially after breast augmentation and tummy tuck surgery. Many patients in this study also reported improvements in self-esteem and a decrease in depression symptoms after their surgery.

Aesthetic facial surgery is designed to make you look younger, but it can also change how people perceive you. An attractive person reveals a heightened self-esteem to the people around them. Women who've had facial rejuvenation are perceived as more likable, attractive, and feminine, and they are believed to have better social skills, as discovered in a study that recorded the responses of people who looked at random photographs.[5]

In the study, subjects were asked to look at several photographs, each of a white female. All the women in the photos had undergone aesthetic facial plastic surgery and a before/after shot was taken. The test subjects only saw either a before or after shot of a woman, not both, to eliminate recall bias. Subjects rated the photographs on six personality traits as well as attractiveness and femininity. The study revealed that rejuvenation of the face and eyes improves a woman's personality as observed by other people. The women were thought to be more likable, had better social skills, and were more attractive and feminine after a facelift.

Women also face pressure in the workplace to look young. A patient of mine who worked as an executive secretary for nearly thirty years was released as she was approaching age fifty. After struggling for a year going through many futile interviews while looking for another executive secretarial position, she decided to have the eyelid surgery that she'd been contemplating for years. Three weeks after her eyelid surgery, she was offered a more lucrative post with a new corporation. The interviewers all commented on her alertness and ideas. She was convinced that her fresh new look and new confidence helped her land the new and better job.

For actors and nationally prominent people, the pressure to look young is especially brutal. It's well-known that younger female actors get more and better parts than older actors. It's this struggle that has encouraged Hollywood to maintain a youthful appearance and seek out plastic surgery interventions. Some female actors have begun to "freshen up" their look as early as age seventeen! A twenty-five-year-old female actor recently told me that she doesn't know anyone in her age group and status who *isn't* doing something to maintain their youthful appearance. Almost all of them have injectables (neuromodulators and fillers), chemical peels, and laser therapies. Surgical interventions include breast, nose, and eye surgery. Most female actors have their noses made smaller in their later teens and liposuction of their "double" chins in their early twenties. This female actor confided that because of the angle at which "selfies" are taken, people could see their chins in a whole new way. Since many felt their chins were inadequate, plastic surgeons saw an increase in requests for chin implants.

Beautiful, "perfect" women are needed in advertisement work because they do little or no acting and are just for the background. These models look great on camera, but they all look the same: flawless skin, narrow noses, full and high cheeks, overdone neuromodulators, hair extensions for long and silky hair, eyelash enhancements, and manicured eyebrows.

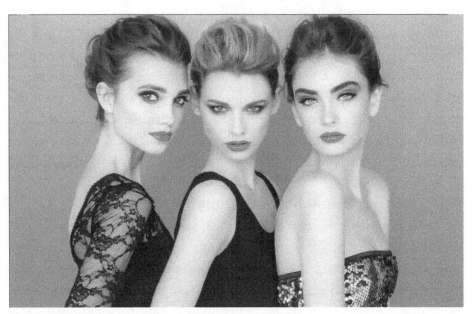

Their flawless, perfect skin with uniform color and no visible pores is the result of extreme laser treatments, deep peels, and overfilling with injectables. The flawless look photographs well and is perfect in a snapshot for the moment. But this look doesn't work for actors. More serious female actors still get skin treatments, injectables, and surgery but often nothing too extreme. These female actors need to show emotion on the set and look like human beings because they're playing real people on the screen.

Perhaps a driving force that couldn't have been predicted has become apparent with the rise of social media. First impressions used to be made in person and influenced with personality as well as appearance. Today, more appearance-driven first impressions are being made on social media—and those images may be digitally manipulated. The use of image-enhancing filters has altered some people's perceptions of attractiveness. While the person may possess the highlighted features, filters can create a look that is unobtainable in real life. The appearance of these digitally manufactured faces is now sought after by many requesting surgery or interventions. The fantasy digital image can lead to lip and cheek injections, nose reductions and chin enhancements, and laser skin treatments to soften the skin texture as well as remove irregular skin colors.

Another unexpected driver came about in 2020 because of Covid-19. The wearing of face masks during the pandemic naturally put the emphasis on the eyes. This has resulted in more requests for neuromodulator injections for eyebrow elevation and the elimination of crow's feet on the outside of the eye and eyelid surgery to remove upper eyelid skin excess and/or puffy lower eyelids. Even simple enhancements like tattoo eyeliner became more commonplace.

Who's Getting Cosmetic Work Done?

As noted at the start of this chapter, about 92 percent of cosmetic patients are females. These patients range from women who undergo only one procedure during their lifetime to almost a third of women who have multiple procedures done to correct aging issues. Most women in the national spotlight are trying to maintain a youthful appearance. This includes successful businesswomen, broadcasters, and politicians. Younger women are more likely to seek improvements for the upper face and eyes, while women over fifty seek surgical corrections of the lower face and neck. Most female professionals choose less image-altering procedures and want only an updated, refreshed look.

This workplace pressure applies to men as well, and in fact, the percentage of men undergoing plastic surgery has increased to about 20 percent in some plastic surgery practices. A simple eyelid surgery done well in a male makes a significant improvement in how they appear to their coworkers and acquaintances. A conservative removal of redundant upper eyelid skin can create a more alert and energetic appearance.

Besides workplace pressure, there's also the social pressure to look fit and attractive. Sometimes this can't be accomplished by working out, making surgical interventions necessary. In a woman, this may include breast reduction or augmentation, liposuction, tummy tuck, and buttock or extremity implants. In the male, it's all about accentuating the muscles and may include liposuction, male breast reduction, and chest or calf implants.

But it's not only the rich and famous getting cosmetic work done. The inflation-adjusted cost of cosmetic surgery today is less than what it was thirty years ago when I started my practice.[6] This cost reduction is because the number of providers has increased and patients can choose their providers based upon a competitive marketplace and price transparency. Choice will always allow the price to drop. It's possible to find qualified providers at a fair price, but good plastic surgery will never be cheap. Finding appropriately educated and experienced providers isn't possible at bargain prices.

Even with the lower cost per procedure, Americans overall are spending more on cosmetic interventions than they were twenty years ago, and it isn't only the wealthy and the famous getting plastic surgery. Published research has shown that the mean household income of over 7,000 patients undergoing 8,000 procedures was $60,976.[7] Breast augmentation claimed the lowest household income per patient at $54,000, while facelift surgery had the highest at $67,000. Only *13 percent* of patients overall had incomes greater than $90,000 a year. Given these lower incomes, many patients save money for years to fund their plastic surgery desires. A recent patient of mine saved frugally for five years to pay for her breast augmentation, breast lift, and tummy tuck. I've seen jars full of small change marked "For my plastic surgery" and even a ceramic "Boob Job Fund" jar.

Increasing Surgical and Nonsurgical Procedures

From 1997 to 2018, the number of surgical procedures doubled. That may sound like a lot (and it is), but consider this. In the same time frame, nonsurgical procedures increased *over ninefold*. These nonsurgical procedures include neuromodulator injections promoted as a "chemical brow lift," artificial fillers described as giving a "liquid facelift," and laser resurfacing promoted as skin "rejuvenation." All these procedures are promoted as simulating or as a substitute for more invasive surgical improvements.

Surgical Procedures

The total number of plastic surgery procedures went from 939,000 in 1997 up to 1.8 million procedures in 2018.[8] Some procedures contribute more to this increase than others. The number of liposuction cases doubled. Breast augmentations increased almost three times and tummy tucks increased almost fivefold. Facial surgery numbers including nose surgery, eyelid lifts, and facelifts remained flat over those years.

All surgical procedures require an incision be made in the skin and range from minimal *closed* procedures to full *open* procedures. Examples of closed procedures include:

- *Liposuction.* This requires small openings to be made in the skin to extract the fat cells.
- *ThreadLift.* Small incisions are made to accommodate the placement of threads under the skin that are used to pull and elevate the underlying tissue structures, thereby giving the face a lift.
- *Endoscopic.* A small incision allows for insertion of an optic instrument (endoscope) to visualize tissue in a large area underneath the skin without a large incision. Endoscopic procedures may provide lift or stretch to the underlying

deeper structures (e.g., endoscopic forehead lift or endo-scopic breast augmentation).

Mini open procedures (mini facelift, mini tummy tuck, and a lim-ited breast lift) that utilize small skin incisions and limited skin removal may have great success in appropriate patients. The classic facelift, tummy tuck, and breast lift procedures are *full, open* operations with significant skin removal and extensive repositioning of deeper structures.

Nonsurgical Procedures

Although the 21st century has seen more people opting for surgical procedures, many new *noninvasive* and *minimally invasive* procedures have been developed over the last decade, giving the public additional options. These less-invasive treatments are advertised as replacements for or enhancements to traditional surgery. These procedures tend to be less expensive, and the patient can resume full activities more quickly.

The overall increase in aesthetic procedures is due mainly to the increasing numbers of office-based nonsurgical procedures, such as injec-tions and laser therapies. The American Society of Plastic Surgeons (ASPS) reported that board-certified plastic surgeons performed almost sixteen million minimally invasive cosmetic procedures in 2018. This number represents a 5,000 percent increase over the last fifteen years.[9] These num-bers don't include procedures performed by other surgeons, physicians, and nonphysician providers.

The ongoing development of noninvasive or minimally invasive proce-dures has increased the number of people seeking cosmetic improvements, although it's also made it possible for people who aren't board-certified plastic surgeons to advertise and perform these procedures. Currently, these nonsurgical procedures are performed five times more frequently than surgical procedures.

I attempt to explain the differences between neuromodulators, facial fillers, lasers, and light therapies to my patients almost every day. Not all injectables are Botox, and not all skin therapies involve lasers. A question that I'm asked repeatedly is, "Do I need Botox or Juvéderm?" The patient may be convinced they need filler when they really need a neuromodulator and vice versa. The only thing neuromodulators and fillers have in common is that a needle is used to inject the material under the skin. Patients will also ask for laser treatments when they really need intense pulse light (IPL) photo-rejuvenation procedures to address skin pigment issues. This isn't surprising! With so many options available, it's no wonder it's so confusing. Unfortunately, some providers' office staffs don't fully understand the differences between options when asked by patients. I hear some crazy stories from patients who come to me after a questionable experience elsewhere.

Noninvasive Procedures

Noninvasive procedures are techniques where the skin isn't violated or pierced. These procedures include external ultrasound and radio-frequency therapy, heat and cold transmission, microcurrent electrical delivery, and visible and non-visible light therapies.

- External ultrasound (US) and radio-frequency (RF) deliver heat to stimulate collagen production and achieve temporary filling, lifting, and tightening.
- Heat and cold external transmission only injure fat cells under the skin to allow the body to self-digest and remove the cells.
- Microcurrent electrical delivery provides a temporary lift by tightening the muscles.
- Light therapies are absorbed through the skin surface, passing to various depths. Visible light can address general redness, veins, rosacea, and pigmentation issues. The blue light visible range travels to the depth of the pore and sebaceous glands of the skin and is useful in controlling acne. It works to destroy the acne bacteria and reduce the oil production inside the pore/sebaceous gland structure.

When the blue light is combined with a topical agent called levulon (PDT-PhotoDynamic Therapy), the intensity of the treatment is increased to treat more severe acne, correct fine wrinkles, and eliminate precancerous lesions of the skin. Non-visible light therapies (infrared) heats and tightens the skin.

Minimally Invasive Procedures

Minimally invasive treatments accomplish more rejuvenation than noninvasive procedures. But these procedures necessitate disruption of the skin's surface. Minimally invasive procedures include neuromodulator injections, filler placement, and laser resurfacing.

The most popular minimally invasive procedures include:

- Neuromodulators that temporarily reduce movement when injected into the muscle. Years of repetitive muscle movement cause wrinkles and lines in the face. The use of neuromodulators suspends the muscle movement, thereby reducing permanent wrinkles.
- Fillers, which are used to refill areas that have been depleted due to aging. Replacing lost volume with either synthetic material or the patient's own fat will temporarily correct loose, wrinkled skin.
- Laser therapies, which are used to resurface the skin to reduce wrinkles and skin discolorations. The surface of the skin is buffed or sanded down to a particular depth that's adjusted by the provider. The depth of the laser treatment and the number of treatments needed depends on the skin damage needing correction, the level of patient pain tolerance, and the amount of time that can be reserved for recovery.

Throughout this book, the use of the term *injectables* means either neuromodulators or fillers that are injected under the skin.

Neuromodulators

As a general rule, neuromodulators (Botox, Xeomin, and Dysport) are used to correct wrinkles resulting from muscle forces on the skin. The Food and Drug Administration (FDA) initially approved Botox for cosmetic uses in 2002. Now, Botox injection is the most commonly performed nonsurgical cosmetic procedure and accounts for half of the nonsurgical procedures performed last year. Over 7.4 million Botox injections were reported in 2018 by board-certified plastic surgeons. This number doesn't include non-board-certified plastic surgeons. The numbers greatly increase when medical physicians, dermatologists, ophthalmologists, and medical spa employees are included.

Neuromodulators are most typically used around the eyes and the forehead. They can lift the brow, open the eyes, and soften the lines of the forehead and around the eyes (crow's feet). Extra care should always be taken if using neuromodulators around the mouth. If used indiscriminately, the patient runs the risk of a crooked smile that can make them look as if they just returned from the dentist or worse, had a recent stroke. The crooked smile is gone in a couple hours after a visit to the dentist, but with neuromodulator injections, it can up to last three to four months before the neuromodulator wears off.

Fillers

The use of fillers has transformed the aesthetic industry by restoring lost volume to the aged, deflated face. Since surgery tightens the skin but poorly restores volume, a combination of moderate skin tightening, along with limited volume restoration using fillers, results in a natural, rejuvenated appearance. Cheeks, lips, and folds around the mouth are commonly filled areas of the face. The thin skin under the eyes with an underlying arcade of blood vessels should be injected with great caution or avoided completely. Only a physician with a lot of experience injecting fillers should inject around the eye because of the risk of blindness if some filler material enters a blood vessel.

The use of synthetic fillers increases every year even as the costs increase. Many types of filler are already available, and more are developed every year. The large companies that service the cosmetic-based medical offices are in a race to develop the best and longest-lasting fillers. How quickly the patient metabolizes particular filler material accounts for some of the difference in material longevity. The commonly used hyaluronic gel fillers (e.g., Restylane and Juviderm) will last for six to twelve months. Some hyaluronic gel fillers (e.g., Restylane Silk and Belotero) are designed to rest close to the skin surface where they fill in very fine lines. These may last as little as six weeks. Some longer-lasting hyaluronic gel fillers (e.g., Restylane Lyft and Voluma) are placed deeper and last one to two years. Mid-depth placement fillers include calcium hydroxyapatite (Radiesse) and poly-L-lactic acid (Sculptra), both of which may last up to two years. A combination product of cow collagen and polymethylmethacrylate microspheres (Bellafill) is marketed as lasting five years.

Fat injections are revolutionizing the filler world and may be a better alternative for use in the face. However, this is an invasive procedure that requires additional downtime since the swelling can be more significant than with synthetic fillers.

Fat survives as a graft from 2 to 98 percent of the time. In my office, we quote a 50 percent survival rate as the average, knowing that some people will have a 2 percent rate and others a 98 percent rate. The patients with a 2 percent survival rate can have more fat injected. But for the over-achieving 98 percenters, they'll look over-injected, now sporting a "trout pout," "pillow face," or a "horse mouth." These results aren't what was intended and give the patient an obvious unnatural look.

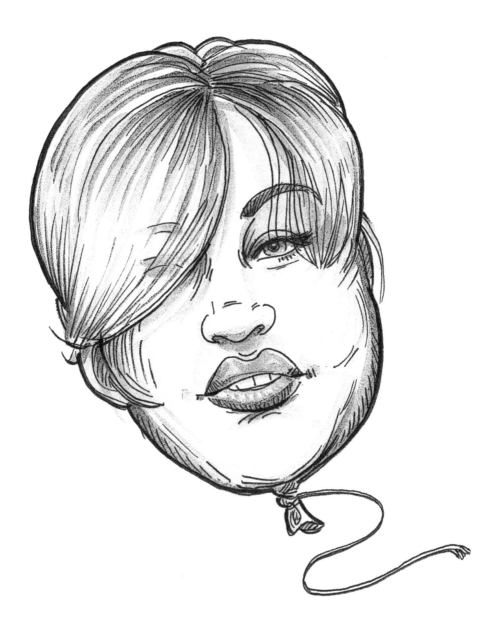

Fat survival rate is also unpredictable in different areas of the face. One area could see a 50 percent survival while another could see an 80 percent rate. The result will be lumps, bumps, or the dreaded "ping pong" face. Unlike synthetic fillers, which go away eventually unless they can be dissolved with an enzyme, fat doesn't go away easily, making these deformities exceedingly difficult to correct. And, while fat injections can provide good results, they don't always last, leaving patients needing synthetic fillers about one year after fat grafting.

Ablative and Nonablative Treatments

Laser therapy frequently comes to mind when people discuss skin rejuvenation. However, a laser (Light Amplification by Stimulated Emission of Radiation) machine is not the only treatment used in nonsurgical skin renewal therapies. Skin rejuvenation can be accomplished using a variety of techniques generally known as ablative and nonablative treatments.

Lasers and peels are *ablative* treatments because they remove layers of skin cells and disrupt the skin surface, requiring a period of downtime and recovery. The extent of the laser treatment and the recovery time depends on the percentage of skin treated and the depth of the injury. Most ablative lasers uniformly remove the top skin cell layers and are recommended to improve fine lines. The surface of the skin is removed down to a programed depth as adjusted into the laser. The skin removal can be superficial, which includes the top layer of skin (epidermis), or just above the junction between the superficial and the deeper areas of skin (the epidermal/dermal junction). Any injury below this junction into the dermis may cause healing problems and scarring. More wrinkles are removed with deeper resurfacing, but a longer recovery is also required for healing.

Fractional lasers remove just a fraction (up to one fifth or 20 percent) of the skin surface and are typically used to penetrate into these deeper layers of skin. The ability to go deeper into the skin is possible with a fractional laser since the laser affects only a small portion (fraction) of the skin surface. The result is similar to the surface of a pegboard or cribbage board with deep holes in the skin, which allows the younger, deeper cells to migrate through the channels/holes to repopulate the skin surface. The fractional laser is especially useful for deep wrinkles and acne scarring.

Chemical peels such as phenol, trichloroacetic acid-TCA, etc. remove the top skin cells by a reaction that disrupts the fats holding the skin cells together. Since the cells can no longer hold themselves together, the cells fall away or "peel" from the skin. The depth of the peel depends upon the chemical used, the percentage of the chemical in the peel solution, and the length of time the chemical is in contact with the skin. The body responds to either laser skin removal or chemical skin peeling by increasing its own repair mechanisms with increased collagen formation, which results in new, healthier, better appearing skin.

The biggest misconception about *ablative* laser therapies or peels is that it requires only one treatment. One intense treatment with a deep laser or peel results in more pain, a longer recovery, and the need to protect the skin while it's healing so scarring can be prevented. The healing process from a raw, exfoliated surface to new skin may take weeks. The healing skin needs special care with anti-inflammatory products, plenty of antioxidant-rich moisturizers, and zinc-based sunscreens. Because of this extended recovery with a deeper skin injury, several superficial laser treatments or peels done at regular intervals are more appealing to most people. The results are cumulative if done with short intervals between treatments.

In comparison, *nonablative* or noninvasive skin therapies go below the skin surface and don't disrupt the overlying skin cells. Typically, no recovery time is required after a procedure, which makes it attractive to many patients. Patients may go out to dinner that evening and experience little downtime from their regular activities. The nonablative energy bypasses the skin surface and works on the deeper tissues. These treatments include light (IPL), heat (RF, ultrasound—US), freezing (cryolipolysis—"fat freezing"), and chemical dissolving (chemolipolysis—"fat dissolving"). The results of these therapies are more subtle and a bit of time needs to pass before obvious changes can be seen.

Less-invasive procedures deliver modest improvements that are shorter lasting than more invasive procedures. The results of most nonablative procedures peak at three months. Unfortunately, most results fade by six months and need to be performed again.

A word of caution: Undergo nonablative, nonsurgical treatments with appropriate expectations of the results. These types of treatments don't give surgical results. About 50 percent of patients are satisfied with the results of their nonablative therapies, but physician satisfaction averages around 30 percent. In contrast, satisfaction after surgery approaches 90 percent for both patient and surgeon.

Because nonablative, noninvasive, and minimally invasive procedures don't involve surgery, they've created a new cosmetic market that's now populated with all sorts of non-surgeon providers. Non-surgeon providers stress the advantage of nonsurgical interventions, but often these procedures are severely overused (e.g., overfilled or motionless faces) and only delay the desire for surgery. Even though promoted as safer, these lesser procedures have their own unique set of complications, especially when delivered by poorly or even untrained personnel. It's quite common for new patients who come into my office for surgery to have already spent almost as much on fillers and neuromodulators as they could have for a facelift.

Chapter 5
Patients with Bad Outcomes

- - - - - - - - - - -

Whether a surgical or nonsurgical treatment, things can go wrong, giving a botched result. Most poor surgical results occur because of poor selection of the procedure or surgeon. Nonsurgical problems occur because the patient is a poor candidate for the procedure or the technical limitations of the chosen procedure.

Patient Problems

Thirty percent of the surgical cases I perform are corrective surgery for bad outcomes of previous plastic and aesthetic surgery. Five of my patients are noteworthy and illustrate the bad plastic surgery I help repair on a regular basis. The names are fictitious but their problems are not.

Frances

Frances was a highly educated specialty physician who came to the office with the complaint of "facial aging issues." As I walked into the exam room to greet her, she stated, "I've spent over twenty-five thousand dollars on gimmicks and am ready to spend that money now on the facelift I should have invested in years ago."

During our subsequent discussion, she confessed to thinking she was doing everything the right way. She didn't want anything extreme that involved downtime, so she sought out lesser procedures and aesthetic physicians. She'd never consulted with a plastic surgeon who could have surgically corrected some of her complaints.

To decide the treatments she thought she needed, Frances did a lot of online research on skin care and procedures. She spent hours reading about each option prior to making her selections. She researched every new technology. She looked at multiple physician websites around the country and critiqued the patient pictures that were displayed. She read the reviews of the physicians and facilities she was considering before making her decision. She felt she was well educated and confident in her choices.

Frances underwent multiple peels, microneedling, Botox and filler injections, laser therapies, ultrasound treatments, and deep heating sessions in the hopes of correcting her aging skin. Most of these treatments were done using different professionals because all the procedures she wanted weren't offered by one provider.

Frances was the only oversight and coordinator for her own care. Not being a plastic surgery professional, she didn't understand the implications of the various treatments. By the time she came to see me, her face was white with a waxy appearance from overdone peels and lasers. All the red or brown pigments in her skin were gone and she had no visible pores. Heat damage caused by deep collagen stimulation treatments had left her with deep indentations in her face due to fat loss. Her face was nearly expressionless and had lost its animation. Her eyes had become small slits due to overfilling her cheeks with fat and fillers. Instead of a soft, doughy feel to her deep tissues, her face had a very unnatural firmness and grittiness due to the deep heat therapies and overstimulation of new collagen.

After my examination, I recommended she wait to have surgery and allow her face to heal and absorb all of the injected material. I explained that I didn't want surgical manipulation to introduce new injuries on top of the injuries she already had. She was unmoved; she wanted corrective surgery right away. I held firm and told her she should wait until the soft tissues had recovered. She listened, and I did her eyelid and facelift surgery two years later.

Gloria

Gloria called the office and asked to be seen on an extremely urgent basis. She'd gone to Mexico to have multiple procedures performed. When she called, it had been about two weeks since her surgery. Her procedures included a tummy tuck, breast augmentation, breast lifts, and liposuction. Gloria called my office because her stomach was swollen and hot, her nipples had turned black, a dark black "thing" was coming out of the right breast incision, and multiple areas on her thighs were draining pus.

I saw her in my office immediately. As I examined her, I saw a large burn on her abdominal wall. She said the doctor told her it was the result of electrocautery malfunction. Further investigation revealed that she had almost a liter of blood in the abdominal surgical site. I drained the blood and cultured it. Multiple cultures were also taken of the drainage coming from her thighs. I had the sad job of informing her that her nipples were dead and necrotic, and the dark, black "thing" coming out of the right breast incision was a breast implant. It was removed and cultured. When the lab returned the culture results, the data showed a rarely seen fungus. She required three subsequent surgeries to correct all the problems.

When I asked why she'd gone to Mexico for her surgery, she admitted it was to save money. She thought she'd done a good job researching her surgeon online but relied on reviews by other patients as the final determiner. There wasn't a presurgery meeting with the surgeon; she only met him the morning of her procedures. After all Gloria has been through, I'm certain that if she could make the decision all over again, she'd never choose a doctor based on the information she found online.

Beth

Beth underwent a "mommy makeover" about two years ago. Her procedure included a tummy tuck, neck liposuction, and breast augmentation with both an implant and fat harvested from her thighs and arms injected into her breasts. Over the last year, she'd gained seventy-five pounds. She called the office because her body just didn't look right anymore after her weight gain. She also told our nurse that she was recently worked up for lymphoma because of a large mass in her neck. Doctors thought it was an enlarged lymph node, but the biopsy showed *fat*.

As I examined her, I noted that her neck was disproportionally small for a somewhat full face. I felt multiple nodules in her neck that easily mimicked lymph nodes. Her upper arms were also small in comparison to her forearms, giving her "Popeye" arms. I detected multiple nodules in her breasts that could be mistaken for cancer nodules. In fact, her last mammogram produced suspicious results and she required further testing. Because of her weight gain, her breasts had enlarged, becoming ptotic (or droopy). Her implants were sitting high on her chest with her now-enlarged breasts hanging and pointing downwards. Her abdominal wall looked "bizarre and weird." The upper abdominal wall and flanks were thick, but her lower abdominal wall was flat with less than an inch to pinch. Her pubis was swollen, and the swelling extended down into her labia.

The previous surgeon must have done liposuction on her buttocks, because with the weight gain, the new fat preferentially deposited along the lower and outer aspects of her buttock, making it appear flat, wide, and square instead of round and projecting.

She didn't like the fact that I suggested she correct the skin excess only after she'd gotten back to her presurgical weight. When I told her that weight gain after liposuction tends to be core fat, which is very unhealthy, she understood the danger and used that as an incentive to lose the weight.

Aaron

Aaron called for an appointment because he looked "weird and sinister" after a recent browlift, facelift, nose, and eyelid surgery. He also revealed over the phone that he had white, semi-soft material coming through the skin on the tip of his nose. He also noted that he had to shave behind his ears and his beard was growing into his ear canal. He stated that he really didn't want to have all these different procedures done, but the surgeon had told him it would give his face more balance if it was all done at once. In fact, Aaron said his nose, although somewhat thick at the tip, didn't bother him at all.

During his appointment, he showed me his driver's license. He didn't look at all like his picture, which was only two years old. It was evident that the brow elevation was too high, especially between the eyebrows, giving him a surprised look at all times. His forehead was motionless. He couldn't completely close his eyes, and they'd been shortened in the transverse plane, making his eyes look "beady and sinister." His facelift was also pulled too tight, which pulled his beard into the ear canal and up behind the ears. The extreme pull subsequently flattened his face. His scars were thickened and noticeable. The material extruding from the tip of his nose was dead nasal tip cartilage.

Over the next two years, we worked together to correct all his issues, starting with the nose and lowering the brow.

Dana

Dana called the office from her car demanding, "Dr. Francel has to see me *now!*" Against medical advice, she had signed herself out from a large local teaching hospital with complications from breast cancer and breast reconstructions. She was diagnosed with right breast cancer and had undergone mastectomies and reconstruction using her own abdominal tissue.

Her first surgery had been seventeen hours long and was followed by another ten-hour surgery five days later for complications. She had spent twenty days in the intensive care unit, requiring twenty-one units of blood. While she was hospitalized after surgery, she had asked everyone who cared for her who they would go to if they had this complication. She left the hospital and came straight to my office. She had large wounds and dead tissue on both breasts and her abdominal wall. I said to her upon seeing these wounds, "Dana, you and I are going to be close friends because of all the time we'll spend together." We're still close friends fifteen surgeries and eighteen years later.

Jeanne

Jeanne came to see me for an embarrassing problem. She saw a non-surgeon physician who performed inner thigh liposuction in his office. After that procedure, her skin was loose and hanging. The surgeon did a thigh lift to "lift" the skin. After the surgery, she complained of perineal dryness problems. Her surgeon talked her into a secondary inner thigh lift, stating that if he took more skin it would correct her dryness. Unfortunately, after this "corrective" surgery, the dryness was worse. She also had a new problem. Air would enter her vagina as she walked and was expelled in a very embarrassing manner. A physical exam revealed that except when she crossed her legs, her labia were pulled apart because of the thigh skin removal. As she walked, her introitus would open, allowing air to enter her vagina and subsequently escape in a loud fashion. I performed corrective surgery on her about a month later.

This chapter serves to introduce these six patients and the problems they encountered. In subsequent chapters, you'll learn more about them, what influenced the decisions they made regarding aesthetic procedures, how they chose their doctors, and what sway the internet and cosmetic product manufacturers had on their decisions. You'll also gain insight into the physicians and other personnel who performed their procedures and better understand the procedures themselves. By the end of the book, you should be able to identify the reasons why these six people had bad plastic surgery.

Bad Plastic Surgery Examples

If you do an online search for "bad plastic surgery," you'll be met with many images of common offenders.

Three people who reliably show up in these searches are Jennifer Grey, Renee Zellweger, and Michael Jackson. In my opinion, none had bad plastic surgery. In fact, the surgeries corrected imbalances that created their distinctive looks, and that's why these three tend to appear on bad plastic surgery lists—they made major changes to a distinctive anatomic characteristic.

In Jennifer Grey's case, it was her longish nose that everyone remembered from the movie "Dirty Dancing." After surgery, her nose is more aesthetic and in better proportion to her face. It fits better into the aesthetic ratios of an attractive face.

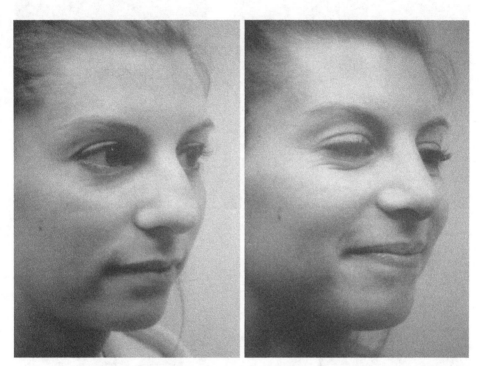

Like Grey, this patient's nose after surgery reveals a better aesthetic of 1.62 to 1.0 of pupil to nasal tip and nasal tip to chin.

But she didn't look like "her" anymore.

Renee Zellweger's trademark appearance was her puffy bedroom eyes that were almost Asian in appearance due to the lack of a well-defined upper eyelid fold. After her surgery, she now has an upper lid crease. The surgery gave her eyes an upper eyelid in the aesthetic one-third to two-thirds ratio of a youthful eye from the lashes to the crease to the eyebrow.

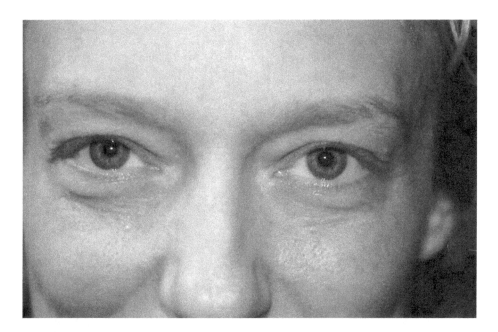

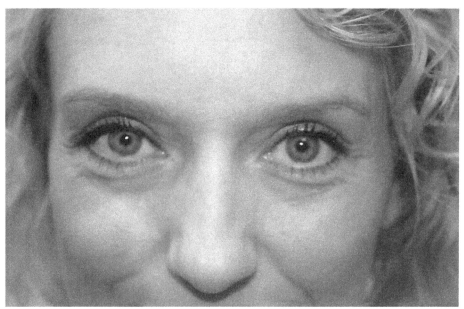

Similar to Zellweger, this patient's postoperative eyes reveal adherence to
the aesthetic ratio of upper lid to eyelid skin crease to lash line instead of her
original full eyelids without a skin crease.

But she no longer looks like "her."

After Michael Jackson's first two nasal surgeries, he had a nose that fit better into the aesthetic ratios: 1) the base and nasal bones were narrowed to better fit the distance between his eyes, 2) the nasal tip was reduced and narrowed to give better tip definition and light reflections, and 3) the nasal dorsum was built up and strengthened.

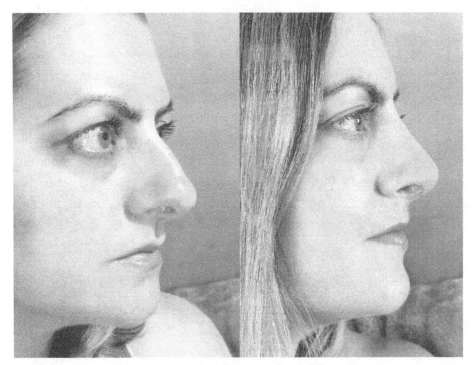

This patient's nose after the first surgeries was narrower both in the mid-portion as well as the base, and the nasal tip was thinner and more defined.

What happened after these initial surgeries added him to the list of bad plastic surgery results. In my opinion, it was the introduction of new nasal procedures, and perhaps even a new surgeon, that led to his nose deteriorating into the frequently criticized and highly controversial "Jackson nose."

The Uncanny Valley

Bad plastic surgery can leave a patient looking less than human. I see this as a big problem. This "not quite human" image is repulsive to most people. When humans see human features on a person, they feel empathy, happiness, and calmness. But when humans see these same features on robots, which appear almost but not quite human, they feel revulsion, distaste, and even fear. In robotics, this inhuman look is termed the "uncanny valley." Animators understand that they can't make the eyes on their characters too realistic or people will feel uncomfortable looking at these "creatures." The feelings suddenly go from cute to creepy. At the bottom of the uncanny valley are zombies.

With surgically altered and overly manipulated faces so prevalent in our society, patients may now be entering the uncanny valley. This is especially true for people wanting to look artificial or plastic (Barbie dolls, etc.) or choosing to adopt animal characteristics. But this also holds true for patients who look odd (e.g., high arching eyebrows), unnatural (e.g., little facial muscle movement), or overly accentuated (e.g., overfilled lips or cheeks).

Patients who have an abundance of noninvasive aesthetic procedures often develop a somewhat strange look. Their skin appears flawless with no lines, no pores, and no pigment. A prominent Beverly Hills dermatologist explained that this appearance is frequently seen in Southern California and is the result of extreme aesthetic interventions.

Skin overworked by lasers and peels loses its brown and red pigments and appears as smooth as porcelain ceramic. The loss of facial lines through the use of neuromodulators and filler injections eliminates shadows and gives the face a polished look. Without lines of demarcation, the facial features blend together. The face loses its unique individual features, creating a waxy-looking face. The overuse of neuromodulators also decreases sweating. This gives the skin an unnatural, buffed appearance without highlights or light reflections. Instead of looking refreshed and natural, these patients look almost dead and embalmed. These zombie lookalikes are at the bottom of the uncanny valley.

With all this bad plastic surgery becoming more common, some feel that we're filling the uncanny valley by showing empathy for these less-than-human-appearing patients. It's as if there's a new fascination with inauthenticity. In fact, some surgeons believe that the future of plastic surgery will be to create a unique or interesting look rather than the present norm of natural or youthful looks. I've had a few patients complain that they look "too natural" after a facelift or eyelid surgery. Some patients want over-accentuated lips, too-full cheeks, and skin as tight as possible.

We're now seeing some people attempting to transform themselves by mimicking celebrities or even taking on animal characteristics. These strange features may become their calling card, and they may soon be described as looking "wonderfully different." It's possible that strange results may one day no longer be considered bad plastic surgery. If that happens, it won't take long for the uncanny valley to be filled.

Chapter 6
Patients Share Responsibility
—Part 1

- - - - - - - - - - - -

J ust as patients share responsibility for their own health (smoking, eating, drinking, drugs, etc.), patients share *some* responsibility for their bad plastic surgery. Our aforementioned patient/physician Frances shared responsibility for her problems when she called my office. I noticed as I walked into a patient room for a new consultation that Frances was sitting next to a large, black garbage bag. Even before I could introduce myself, she pointed to the black bag and said, "I figured it out. I've spent over twenty thousand dollars on this bag of gadgets and creams and none of it works. I'm now here to spend whatever I need to get the results that I have been trying to get with these 'next greatest things' I've used over the last five years."

Inside the bag were an assortment of muscle stimulators, nighttime devices, magnets, and jars of miracle creams that promised surgical results. She had the look of someone who'd done a lot of nonsurgical facial rejuvenation, including thin, colorless, waxy skin, overfilled and ballooning cheeks and mouth, a loss of the defining borders of the aesthetic units of her face, and contour deformities resulting from fillers and heat applications for collagen production.

After we did her eyelid and facelift surgery, she did indeed agree that surgery gave her the result that she'd been seeking. While she thought she was doing everything right by working as her own consultant and choosing to use the less-invasive gadgets, gizmos, and creams, she finally understood that surgical results can only be gained by having surgery.

While Frances finally achieved her aesthetic goals by having plastic surgery, how is it that other patients succumb to "bad plastic surgery"? The reasons I see people ending up with bad plastic surgery fall into four main areas:

1. *Imposing financial and/or time limitations*—choosing a physician or procedure based on price alone or provider availability.
2. *Relying on advertisements, media, and the internet*—learning about procedures only from ads and other paid media versus researching unbiased sources.
3. *Depending solely on physician rating sites or social media presence*—choosing a physician without fully understanding their qualifications or expertise.
4. *Not seeing the big picture of their overall appearance, pursuing skewed aesthetics, or harboring unrealistic expectations of what can be done*—nitpicking on minor issues or wanting a result that's wholly inappropriate or impossible to attain in a natural-looking way.

Imposing Financial and/or Time Limitations

Many prospective plastic surgery patients will save for years to achieve their dream surgery, yet others will pursue their goal of plastic surgery by seeking the least expensive option. Plastic surgery is one place where cheap can be dangerous, more costly than anticipated, and even deadly.

Low Price

Some plastic surgeons offer advertised specials. Beware, as these typically have hidden costs. Cheap breast augmentation typically doesn't include the cost of implants, anesthesia fees, or operating room fees. If the price is all inclusive, you won't be able to tell where these implants were manufactured or if they're FDA approved. The person performing the procedure is trying to make money, so they must be cutting corners somewhere if they're offering plastic surgery at dirt-cheap prices. Are the providers using a cheap surgical facility where they have no emergency equipment, or are they using discounted implants and cheaper surgical supplies? Are they even plastic surgeons? These cheaper surgeries often don't provide appropriate postoperative care. If complications arise, there may be extra charges or you may have to seek out a more experienced surgeon.

Sometimes plastic surgeons use a lower price to gain experience in a particular procedure they see as more profitable. A plastic surgeon in a Midwest city did a lot of reconstructive surgery but wanted to be known as a "facelift surgeon." He undercut the local surgeons by charging only $1,000 for a $7,000 to $10,000 procedure. Unfortunately for his patients, the results weren't good. Many of his patients required expensive secondary surgeries by the more experienced surgeons in the city. Discounted plastic surgery may end up costing more in time and money if additional surgeries are needed.

Free Plastic Surgery

Do you know what's better than cheap plastic surgery? Free plastic surgery!

Several years ago, I received a mass email, which I'm sure went to many plastic surgeons. I give this patient kudos for creativity and the moxie to even ask:

Name: Pearl
Sent: Thursday, May 10, 2007, 1:34 a.m.
Phone: 818-xxx-xxxx
Procedure: breast implants

Dear Doctor: I know this is a lot to ask for but I am not happy about my breasts and I was wondering if you could help me get one for free, please. It will help me a lot since I want to model and they always tell me my boobs are too small. Please help me!

It was obvious that she didn't care who did the surgery or where it was performed, only that it could be done free. I often wonder if anyone took her up on her request.

There are other avenues to getting free plastic surgery.

An article in a tabloid magazine years ago was headlined, "Plastic Surgery for Free." It correctly pointed out that plastic surgeons typically offer their office staff plastic surgery procedures at discounted rates and sometimes even at no charge.

The article pointed out that normally it's required that an employee work for a surgeon for at least one year before undergoing surgery. But surgeons often overlook this requirement—and not for altruistic reasons most of the time either. The surgeon has a living, breathing example of his work right in his office for all prospective patients to see and even possibly touch. Because the staff member has been a patient, the prospective patient feels they're getting the straight scoop about the procedure and all it entails. Unfortunately, staff members often leave after their surgery, presumably because they took the job only for the chance to get free plastic surgery.

It's worth mentioning that this free procedure also carries some risk to the employee. The surgeon can try the newest and greatest procedure on someone other than a potentially litigious patient. Then, if things don't go well, the surgeon can move or remove the staff member so potential patients don't see the poor result in the doctor's office. A plastic surgeon in Maryland did just that. He performed a new nasal procedure on a willing staff member who just happened to be the front office receptionist. After multiple revision surgeries to correct problems, he found the employee a "better job in a nonmedical office" because he couldn't stand looking at the poor result every day and didn't want prospective nasal surgery patients to see her.

You don't have to work in a plastic surgeon's office to get free plastic surgery, though. Instead, you could marry a plastic surgeon. Some of the worst plastic surgery results are seen in plastic surgeons' partners because they're commonly a "guinea pig" for new and innovative procedures. Unfortunately, if a poor result is the outcome, the relationship may not survive because the plastic surgeon can't tolerate looking at a poor result every day *and* night.

If working at a plastic surgeon's office or marrying a plastic surgeon aren't options, some people jump at a chance procedure. Raffles can be held by cities, radio stations, or charities. Winning one of these raffles gives the patient *no choice* in the surgeon providing the procedure (usually a breast augmentation or facelift). Also, the surgeon has no choice in the patient, who might not be a good candidate for the raffled surgery. In all probability, the surgeon supplying the service for the raffle isn't a member of the ASPS because rules and ethics of that society state that members can't operate on raffle winners because neither the surgeon nor the winner has a choice. It's more likely the surgeon offering the services for the raffle is a member of a medical board that's not recognized. Don't participate in these raffles if you want to avoid bad plastic surgery.

Gaming the System with Discounted Injectables

The neuromodulators presently on the market cost over five hundred dollars per vial. If a provider is charging a ridiculously low price for its use, it's either a scheme to get patients in for other services or something other than an FDA-approved neuromodulator—a knockoff.

Sadly, these knockoffs are more common than you'd think. In 2012, the FDA warned many medical practices that the "Botox" received from a Canadian pharmacy was unapproved and could be unsafe.[10] Another later notice warned of a "bogus Botox" being distributed in the United States.[11]

If these unsafe fakes are actually used, the consequences can be dire. This happened in a St. Louis "medical clinic" that purchased more than fifty misbranded "Botox" vials over a two-year period from an unlicensed foreign drug wholesale company. The clinic manager pled guilty to felony charges of receiving drugs from the foreign drug wholesaler. A physician in Florida used a lab-grade neuromodulator used in animal experiments on a number of patients because it was cheaper. Not only was it cheaper, but it was also about one thousand times stronger than what the physician was accustomed to using. All the patients he injected had severe complications. Not all survived.

Even if the neuromodulator is genuine, sometimes physicians are driven by potential profits versus patient outcomes. The practice of diluting a neuromodulator with more fluid than suggested is not uncommon. One diluted bottle can be used to treat more patients at a lower cost to the injector, meaning profits. All the patient receives is a less-than-optimal result.

Finally, inserting or injecting products never designed to be used in the human body is a dark practice in cheap plastic surgery. Many non-approved types of filler have been employed as cost-cutting measures. These products include cooking oil injected into the face, long silk threads passed into the lips, and household silicone inserted into the breast. Almost everything imaginable has been injected to enhance the buttocks, including household caulking compounds, beeswax, mineral oil, cement, Krazy Glue, and motor oil.

A provider of cut-rate buttock injections used a combination of Fix-a-Flat, cement, and Super Glue. Other popular combinations include liquid nonmedical-grade silicone and Super Glue. I evaluated a patient who'd had spray foam insulation injected into her buttock with the promise "It will get bigger overnight" as the spray insulation expanded.

Cut-rate plastic surgery just isn't worth the risks involved just to avoid the extra costs associated with surgeons' fees, anesthesia, and operating room expenses. *Please don't do it.*

Can You Do It Next Thursday?

Some patients seem not so interested in *who does* the surgery or *how much* the surgery costs, but *when* the surgery can be done. A patient came to my office for a breast consultation. My staff and I spent over 90 minutes evaluating her, educating her and her husband, and going over the surgery, including the risks and complications. She called the next day to tell us that she had to have the surgery done next Friday. My operating room schedule was full, so she chose a less experienced surgeon, who was just out of training, because he was open on the day she requested. The surgeon's experience didn't matter; she just wanted the surgery done on the following Friday. Months later, she came in for revision surgery.

Having a "sales and bargains" mentality shouldn't be a consideration when contemplating plastic surgery because it only promotes bad plastic surgery. Qualified plastic surgeons are more expensive, but the improved quality of care and safety are more than worth the extra cost.

However, if you do buy knockoff plastic surgery and then have problems, don't go back to the provider who messed you up as it's likely they won't be able to fix the problems they created. Any complications need to be evaluated and cared for by a qualified, board-certified plastic surgeon.

Needing It for that Big Event

Big events, including weddings, vacations, and high school reunions, are often the impetus that nudges someone toward plastic surgery. I call it "plastic surgery for the moment." Much like a photograph that captures an instant in time and freezes it for posterity, those who seek plastic surgery for a big event are hoping to look great in those photographic memories.

The "Big Event" requests have become so common that I now ask it of every patient that I see. It's better to know the intent of the patient and talk them out of it if they want something drastic (especially with injectables) too close to their big event.

I learned the hard way to ask that question after an established patient of mine came in on a Tuesday to have filler injected for a big national event on Saturday. She needed that filler "for the moment," and that moment was the event Saturday night. I thought I had enough time to manipulate the filler if the injection wasn't just right prior to the event. What I didn't expect was the bruising she developed that was so severe it looked like a "Fu Manchu" beard. She subsequently had to come in every day before the event so we could progressively work with lasers and makeup to cover up the bruising. After that experience, I now require patients to come in at least seven—and preferably ten—days before an event to provide enough time for the initial swelling and bruising to resolve. The same holds true for neuromodulators, lasers, and peels.

For a future bride, a big wedding and all the parties may push her to consider changes to her face and body. What they fail to understand is that there are positives and negatives when choosing plastic surgery "for the moment."

I Want to Look Good Now!

Sometimes there isn't a specific event, just a yearning to look good immediately. Today, many young people see neuromodulator injections as a modern-day status symbol similar to the latest designer clothes, shoes, and purses. Although some use neuromodulators for wrinkles that result from squinting at computer screens and for headaches, many expect these injections to prevent wrinkles in the future. These savvy teens and twenty-somethings also know that regular use of neuromodulators weakens muscles, which decreases the wrinkles associated with repetitive muscle movements. Their goal in continuing to use neuromodulators is to minimize the muscle forces that create new wrinkles and slow the formation of large creases in any existing wrinkles.

The interesting thing about neuromodulators is that they provide instant gratification. But their overuse can border on bad plastic surgery. Having no facial movements can be disturbing to the viewer and borders on the "uncanny valley." Artificial fillers used in the extreme to emphasize a specific area can distort the fine aesthetic points, giving less-than-aesthetic results. Examples of overuse include the "trout pout," which occurs when the lips are overinflated, and the "pillow face," which occurs when the cheeks (and sometimes the whole face) are overinflated.

Look Youthful—or Else

Others may be nudged by their jobs to continue to look youthful to sustain their marketability. Television or movie personnel want to look as young as possible for as long as possible. Keeping their job likely depends on it.

Sometimes people go a little too far to hold on to that youthful visage. A prominent local newscaster had had so much neurotoxin injected in her forehead that she couldn't raise her eyes to look into the camera. She had to raise her head intermittently to look directly into the camera, which meant she couldn't read her script on the table. But her forehead did not have a wrinkle when looking into the camera!

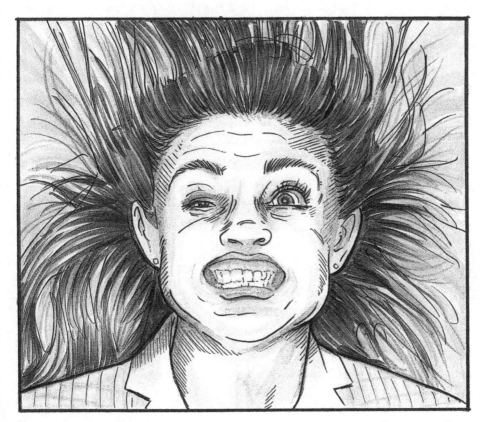

Because celebrities are keen to continue working, it's uncommon for those over age thirty-five to have wrinkles on their faces. This leads the public to believe that the lack of wrinkles on the forehead and around the eyes is youthful and beautiful. It can also lead to people (women especially) to unfairly compare their looks to those of their favorite actors without taking into consideration how much money, time, and effort the actors have spent to look flawless. And, as mentioned earlier, the overuse of neuromodulator injections virtually eliminates the ability to show emotions. A good example of this loss is in the various *Housewives* television shows. These women have had so much done that, even when they're angry with one another, the audience only realizes it because of their raised voices. The full impact of their anger is lost because their foreheads and eyes don't change with their emotions. Imagine the audience's disconnect with an actor showing no facial emotions while lamenting the death of their "child" (Elizabeth Taylor in *Who's Afraid of Virginia Woolf?*).

The Chance of a Lifetime

The world of modeling is brutal, and it's no wonder that even models in their teens will undergo plastic surgery to get into or stay in the modeling game. In the case of a model, getting a big break for a much-coveted photo shoot may be the catalyst. Many young models will have neuromodulator or fillers injected for an upcoming shoot to eliminate forehead and eye wrinkles and plump up their lips. They're chasing the youthful aesthetic, and injections can help keep their eyebrows arched and the upper eyelids full. In image after image, the models' eyebrows haven't changed position even after five hours under the lights. But there's a downside to these injections. Once the models are finished with the shoot, they can't squint to shield their eyes from the sun or raise their eyebrows to indicate surprise or some other emotion.

Another area where models often opt for plastic surgery is the breasts. I've worked with many models who wanted breast augmentation so they could better wear the clothes they'd been hired to exhibit. They often make this decision in the moment for a particular job. They elect to adopt a less natural look to accentuate the clothes, but this look doesn't really fit their body proportions. These models are usually slim, and the D-cup implant they request borders on bad plastic surgery. Many eventually regret their decision and come in later for smaller implants and breast lifts to take up the extra breast skin from the large implants.

I Don't Care What It Takes; I Want It!

Women of all ages will decide they want an invasive procedure, often without a lot of research to understand the long-term consequences of surgical procedures or having foreign substances placed inside the body.

I rarely place breast implants in patients less than twenty years old because they really haven't thought about the life commitment required as an owner. Most of the adolescent females I consult with for cosmetic breast enhancement are looking for the gratification in the moment. I've had prospective patients admit wanting to get breast implants because "My friend had it done" or "It's a graduation present." One patient actually told me that she wanted breast implants for "spring break in Mexico." I'm sure she found another plastic surgeon to fulfill her wish.

Liposuction can be seen as a quick fix to unsightly lumps and bumps, especially before a big event. But far too often, these patients aren't at their ideal weight when requesting this procedure. Worse, many believe they can use liposuction for weight control.

To be clear, liposuction takes away fat cells from specific areas of the body. That doesn't mean the person undergoing a liposuction procedure is guaranteed to stay thinner forever. In fact, if the patient can't lose weight with diet and exercise, she'll probably gain even more weight once her body fat is reduced by liposuction. This weight gain typically happens within the first six to twelve months after the procedure, and it's often significant enough that the patient will complain that the liposuction didn't work. This is what happened with my patient, Beth, who gained seventy-five pounds after her "mommy makeover," leaving her with severe body contour deformities and lumps suggestive of cancer in her neck and breasts.

Since liposuction areas don't have as many fat cells after surgery, any added weight will manifest in other body areas where fat cells are still present, making those areas disproportionately larger than the areas where the fat was suctioned out and removed. For example, after undergoing liposuction of the outer thigh (saddlebag) area, a twenty-pound weight gain will deposit in the inner and front thighs. The saddlebag area, despite having most fat cells removed (it's impossible to remove all of them), will become lumpy because the remaining residual fat cells will still grow. Evidence also supports the fact that some of the fat deposited with weight gain after liposuction ends up as internal or core fat. This gives the patient a new worry as core fat is related to greater health concerns.

What most patients don't realize is that the final result after liposuction is revealed in six months, not six days or even six weeks, which makes it a terrible choice for events happening earlier than six months. I had a patient ask for neck liposuction two months prior to her wedding. I politely refused, pointing out that she wouldn't get the best results in time for the wedding and any complication would be disastrous. Undaunted, she found another surgeon to perform the liposuction surgery.

The result *was* disastrous. In addition to a very swollen neck, she also developed neuropraxia (temporary injury of a nerve) of the main nerve going to the muscles of her face. Needless to say, every wedding picture had a crooked smile on the bride, looking similar to Bell's palsy or a stroke. The damage eventually resolved, but not until well after she'd returned from her honeymoon. Six months after her surgery, you could appreciate the final result.

Relying on Advertisements, Media, and the Internet

The media, including the internet, is often filled with incomplete truths, half-lies, and sometimes outright lies regarding results from skin care, devices, and surgery to modify your looks. Don't use these information sources exclusively when researching your options.

The Miracle Cure

Not all product and equipment manufacturers in the aesthetic industry are out to profit from unrealistic expectations. However, many of these companies offer promises they simply can't keep and people fall for them because they sound so good and seem so easy.

We've all seen and read advertisements like the one below:

> "Avoid painful and risky surgery. Tone and lift your face in five minutes with our incredible new machine employing the energy of _____ to obtain surgical results without the costs, risks, or recovery time of surgery."

Usually attached to the advertisement are fantastic and unbelievable pictures showing incredible and improbable results after using the new equipment, product, or technique. Patients spend tons of time and money in pursuit of the miracle cure that will turn back the clock without undergoing *surgery*. (Remember Frances?)

The pursuit of the miracle cure is what encourages people to buy the newest innovations in aesthetic procedures. Oprah-like television shows survive by promoting "the next greatest thing." These shows make new topical applications or rejuvenation equipment seem like the answer to all your aging concerns. They market directly to the public by "informing and educating" you on what you need to correct your aging features. In this way, they expect you to bypass the advice, experience, and knowledge of your physician. You may have to even inform and educate your physician on what you think is best for you—even if it isn't reality.

These companies studied the success of the pharmaceutical industry. Back in the 1990s, pharmaceutical companies were finally allowed to do "direct-to-consumer" advertising. Prior to this ruling, drug companies relied on doctors to educate their patients. With this change in advertising rules, pharmaceutical companies could take their message straight to consumers. Research has shown that direct-to-consumer prescription drug advertisements increase the sales of the drug. Research also shows that the people who'd most benefit from the drugs aren't the ones securing the prescriptions. The ones getting the drugs are the people who go to their physicians demanding this or that drug they saw advertised on television.

With all the advertisements for aesthetic procedures bombarding the airwaves and the internet and magazines, it's no wonder so many patients come into my office requesting a certain procedure or laser treatment! Just because they saw a wonderful result on a television show or infomercial doesn't mean they're a good candidate for that particular procedure. Usually they're not, and I'm put in the position of explaining the reasons why to the disappointed patient.

The truth is, most of the advertised and/or hyped equipment or procedures aren't better or safer than previous techniques available for giving a cosmetic improvement. The ThreadLift was a cheap alternative to a surgical facelift. The technique was largely abandoned in the 1970s only to be resurrected with disastrous results at the start of this century. This "new" procedure was advertised on television and in magazines as revolutionary and extraordinary but wasn't either. Inexperienced physicians put the threads in, but experienced plastic surgeons had to remove the threads and correct the resulting deformities. The ThreadLift is coming around again, and this resurrection uses absorbable sutures which supposedly "lift and stimulate" soft-tissue growth—but the results only last one year.

Patients need to understand that if it sounds too good to be true, it is. Here are just three examples:

1. Less than a year after a beauty magazine proclaimed a nonsurgical lower eyelid tightener and eye-bag eraser as the "Best of the Beauty Breakthroughs," the eye cream was removed from the marketplace and no longer manufactured presumably because of its ineffectiveness.

2. A manufacturer promoted a "revolutionary technology" that was 100 percent safe and painless. It promised "proven superior clinical results" and was to be used to "reduce cellulite, reduce stretch marks, tighten loose skin, reduce thigh and arm circumference,

reduce wrinkles, reduce swelling, soften lines, and lift tissue for a better shape everywhere on the body." Two years later, the equipment was no longer available because of extensive skin burns.

3. A board-certified plastic surgeon in Missouri offered "exclusive" technology in their office that promised a "noninvasive tummy tuck that involved no general anesthesia, no downtime, no multiple visits, minimal incisions done under local anesthesia, and immediate fabulous results." If such technology actually existed, every provider would invest in that innovative equipment and have it in their office! But that surgeon was the only "exclusive provider" according to his advertisements.

Many patients, disappointed with their results from the less-invasive procedures they've spent hundreds to thousands of dollars on, come to see me eventually to have the appropriate restorative surgery.

Offering the "Latest and Greatest"

Many providers have a narrow vision of the aesthetic industry. They believe to get more patients into their facility, they must have the "greatest and the latest" innovative products, equipment, or technique. Unfortunately, many potential patients are attracted by this narrow vision and no longer make decisions based on service, experience, and results.

Dr. Oz is a surgeon at Columbia College of Physicians and Surgeons in New York City, and in surgical circles, he is a well-respected heart transplant surgeon. He knows a great deal about the heart and how to treat it. But he knows little about skin care, cosmetic devices, or plastic surgery. Yet, during his TV shows, he talks up aesthetic products that have little or no science to support their exaggerated claims, and many of the products he promotes have no clear evidence of benefits. He's just repeating what the advertisers are conveying to him.

A physician in one specialty typically knows little about another specialty. Doctors who aren't trained in plastic surgery are no more knowledgeable about cosmetic procedures than the general public.

One year at a plastic surgery meeting in New York City, a speaker presented results from a new nonablative machine he was using. An astute surgeon in the audience noted that during the same conference the prior year, this same speaker had presented data on a similar machine. The surgeon asked the speaker if he still used the previous modality that he'd presented that provided such brilliant results the year before. The speaker answered no, saying that machine didn't perform as well in his hands as suggested in his first presentation because he was basing it on data supplied by the manufacturer. He concluded that he now uses this new "latest and greatest" machine—and everyone needs to rush out and get one. I saw many in the audience shake their heads, perhaps in disagreement or disbelief.

Physicians will push procedures for profit even if a modality isn't quite right for the patient. Ablative lasers, which replace cheaper chemical peels, cost over $100,000. Nonablative skin machines were introduced to replace the downtime associated with surgical procedures. These machines are marketed as the "latest and the best" and claim fabulous results. When physicians spend this kind of money on one type of machine, they need to promote it as "the next great thing" in order to get a return on their expensive equipment purchase.

There's a risk promoting innovative equipment or procedures. In the world of broken promises, the provider may make money in the short term, but over time, the provider's reputation may suffer. The equipment or procedure may bring in some patients because of national or local advertisements, but the physician's reputation is at risk if this "next great thing" doesn't deliver the results as promised. The reality is that only 10 percent of these great things work as advertised and produce the results as promised. The other 90 percent can tarnish a provider's reputation. In the case of an established surgeon, it may be difficult to separate what he does well from his failures with the latest and greatest technology.

Years ago, I was experimenting with some new technology. A patient advised me, "Stick with what you do best, and that is surgery!" after she saw this new equipment in the office. I listened to her advice and stayed away from unproven procedures and technologies. Having been disappointed many times, I wait for hard, supportive data from real patients in real studies which conform to appropriate and established scientific methods before purchasing a machine. These latest and greatest new therapies generally aren't supported by rigorous scientific methodology, which takes years to acquire. I also no longer take what sales representatives say at face value, as they're simply repeating what they were told by the manufacturer of the equipment.

Sometimes practitioners knowingly lend their name to products and technologies without even having tried them. These next three examples should give you pause.

In 2014, a warning was issued to the plastic surgery community by the editor of a plastic surgery journal (*Plastic Surgery Practice*, May 2014). She'd received an article to review for publication that came from a legitimate plastic surgeon through the surgeon's marketing director. The manuscript detailed some great results from a new piece of equipment. As the editor pushed for more information, it was revealed that the doctor had never actually used the equipment being promoted in the article. Worse, the preoperative and postoperative photographs had been taken from another website. When the editor objected, the marketing director said that it really didn't matter since the article was only meant to be informative, plus it would gain backlinks and boost search engine optimization (SEO) for everyone. The article was not published in this journal.

Years ago, another plastic surgeon published an article in a local newspaper outlining his use of the new ultrasonic liposuction on fifty patients who had no complications and were happy with their results. I was intrigued and called his office to ask him some questions about his experience. Instead of letting me talk with the doctor, his office directed me to the local sales representative of the equipment. The representative confided to me that the surgeon had only used the equipment on ten patients. When I asked about the number discrepancy, he couldn't explain why the article reported the surgeon's results were from fifty patients.

Another plastic surgeon disseminated a press release to local news stations claiming to be "a world-recognized authority in cohesive gel implants…with wide experience and long-term follow-up." His news release said he was "the best," especially at breast implants for augmentation/lift in the massive weight loss patient. Another local plastic surgeon reported him to the National Plastic Surgery Society, and this physician had the dubious distinction of having his many ethics violations cited in a restricted yearly report by the ASPS. Despite his advertising claims, the reality of his experience was that he'd only done three or four implants and his results were far too short to know how they'd turn out. It is obvious he was no expert and exaggerated his experience and ability.

The three plastic surgeons described above violated the American Society of Plastic Surgery Code of Ethics by "using any form of public communication containing a false, fraudulent, deceptive, or misleading statement or claim…which…is intended or is likely to attract patients by use of exaggerated claims." There's really no excuse to market false information just to promote the "next best thing," yet many providers do just that. Unfortunately, no governing body oversees non-board-certified providers, which gives them the opportunity to submit fraudulent claims about their abilities and results.

Shady advertising practices by manufacturers and physicians lead patients down wrong and dangerous roads. Entrusting your face and body to a board-certified plastic surgeon is the best way to avoid results you don't want.

Were You Listening?

Of course, the best plastic surgeon in the world won't be able to help patients who don't listen to what the surgeon is saying. Patients arrive at my office with varying degrees of knowledge. Some have thought long and hard about the surgery they want to have and have done research on the internet to learn as much as they can about a procedure. Others do little research but still have strong opinions about which procedure they believe should be done. Usually their information is from a friend or an advertisement that has convinced them a particular procedure is the right one for them.

Regardless of where the information comes from, the majority of these patients still arrive for their initial consultations confused and bringing with them lots of ideas, expectations, and questions. My job as a plastic surgeon is to educate and instruct my patients. I can explain how the ideas gleaned from their research may not be the right thing for them or how their friend's surgery may or may not be the right surgery for them. Yet even after answering all their questions explaining the procedure, few patients leave completely understanding what was just discussed. What's going on?

Patients don't hear what they don't want to hear. This includes the procedure, the risks and complications, the unintended consequences, and the expected results and outcome. After an initial consultation with one patient, I asked if she had any questions. She then pulled three typed pages of questions out of her purse that she had gotten off the internet entitled, "Questions to Ask Your Plastic Surgeon." I realized after the first four questions that she wasn't really hearing the answers. My answer to her fifth question was, "We already discussed that and I answered that question." She didn't even pause as she asked question number six. My answer to that question was, "We aren't going through all those questions without you hearing me." Again, without hesitation, she proceeded onto question number seven. My answer to that question was, "You are neither listening nor hearing," and then I rose to leave the room. She looked up, startled. I sat down and then tried to help her understand what had just happened and why it was important for her to hear what I was saying.

But not all patients listen or understand even when the information is in writing. A patient came in weeks after a chemical peel with some late healing areas. I asked whether she'd picked at them even though she'd been instructed not to pick her skin in her pre-peel instructions. She responded, "Of course I picked them; they were itchy." Not listening can lead to an unhappy patient and a frustrated surgeon.

Men don't listen any better than women do when it comes to plastic surgery. I once had a 40-year-old male come in to discuss getting a facelift. We spoke about the pros and the cons, but the one thing that I really didn't think he would find acceptable would be the scars. Scars on young men look sexy anywhere except behind the ears. He said that the scars would be fine, but since he was recently single, I felt that he'd have a hard time explaining facelift scars to the new people he was meeting while dating. I passed on doing his surgery. I thought I'd convinced him not to do the facelift only to have him come back to my office two years later after having the procedure done by someone else. He returned to me because of the scars. He said they were noticeable soon after surgery. He wanted to have something done right away to correct them, so the surgeon who'd done the surgery tried an early surgical correction. They didn't improve. The surgeon then attempted to correct them with laser therapy, which only made the scars worse and more noticeable. I shook my head and wished he'd listened to my advice years ago. Now there were few options available to correct his problem.

The problem of not listening was highlighted in a small study conducted by a plastic surgeon. At this surgeon's office, an employee sat in the waiting room with a laptop and asked the patient what questions they had for the doctor before their appointment. The employee recorded this information and gave the list to both the patient and the doctor. When the consultation was over, the patient was asked to complete the answers to their questions. The patient's answers only corresponded 20 percent of the time with what the doctor said. Because I want my patients to be fully informed and understand what they're about to do, I always ask them to come in for a second visit about two weeks prior to their surgery. During this visit, we may again go over all their concerns and questions. I encourage them to bring in a spouse, relative, or friend to be a second independent set of ears and who can write down the answers to the patient's questions for later review.

Doing your own research is great, but just don't let it be your only source for information. Listen to and depend upon your plastic surgeon to fully understand the procedure you're about to undergo.

Depending Solely on Physician Ratings Sites

Frances, Aaron, and Jeanne thought they were doing the right thing by choosing their providers based on their extensive review of online physician rating sites. Plastic surgeons used to be rated by their *visual results* and *postoperative patient satisfaction*. Today, rating sites claim to be the best indicator of who's a good practitioner and who's not. Unfortunately, online reviews of plastic surgeons tend to be *unreliable*. And that's putting it nicely.

These rating sites poorly evaluate a surgeon's training, knowledge, and technical skills. Worse, you can't learn from a rating site how dedicated a surgeon is to their patients, their level of empathy, or their ability to listen to each individual's concerns.

Positive physician rating sites don't predict better outcomes, and data actually suggests that patient satisfaction and surgical outcomes don't even correlate. A review from Northwestern University in Chicago showed that it's difficult for consumers to obtain good, balanced information about a surgeon's *results*—the most important metric by which to evaluate a plastic surgeon—from online rating sites.

The Northwestern University study reviewed ratings by patients who may or may not have consulted the provider or may or may not have had surgery with that plastic surgeon.[12] Important factors in these ratings included how quickly the phone is picked up, how "nicely" the staff responds, and the wait times to be seen by the physician. Other factors included the office environment, punctuality, helpfulness, bedside manner, and costs. All these factors can be evaluated without ever having a procedure performed by that plastic surgeon. These sites don't rate a surgeon's experience, ability, or results. Service seems to be more important than visible results and outcomes.

Using these sites as your only determiner as to whether to use a physician or not is a mistake. The reality is that the best surgeons will be fully booked, have longer wait times, and won't have the time to sit and ask for your family medical history. They'll also have a busier and more stressed staff.

Probably one of the best and most renowned, among his peers, plastic surgeons struggled with poor online ratings. He frequently traveled to educate his colleagues, which meant long appointment wait times. He was frequently called out of a patient's consult to help another plastic surgeon calling from a distant operating room asking for advice with a surgery. He was the editor of a major aesthetic plastic surgery journal that required long hours even after late office hours. On top of all that, he was a professor of surgery who lectured and taught plastic surgery trainees. Even though he was one of the best in the world, his ratings were stuck in the middle of the one to five rating scale used on physician rating sites. But wouldn't you rather have this *renowned* plastic surgeon operating on you in a *certified surgical facility* in two months versus going to a surgeon whose staff was nice, who gave you an appointment that week, and could schedule you for surgery the next week in a *noncertified in-office* operating room?

The ratings on these sites are easily manipulated by the person being rated as well as by competitors who attempt to make a physician look bad. Knowledgeable consumers typically and appropriately dismiss an anonymous negative review as an attempt by a jealous competitor or a disgruntled employee to berate a successful surgeon. An excellent board-certified plastic surgeon was declared "a butcher" by a "patient" on a ratings website. It turned out the "patient" was a mother who was upset that the surgeon did a breast augmentation on her twenty-five-year-old daughter. The daughter was thrilled with her result.

Dubious reviews are common and sometimes hard to spot. In the case of the next four examples, the bogus ratings are obvious:

- A doctor in Florida had his license permanently revoked, but his office was still receiving online evaluations one year later. Reviews such as "Best doctor in town" and "Couldn't be happier with results" were posted. And this one appeared two years after he lost his license: "I highly recommend this doctor." One rating website still rates him three out of four stars years later!

- A Brooklyn doctor pled guilty in a liposuction patient's death. Months later, he received an online "Patient's Choice Physician Award" for "the quality of care and service he provides." His record also included three previous complaints for professional misconduct, substandard care, and incompetence or neglect.
- A Boston cosmetic surgeon had his license revoked for failure to maintain professional boundaries with patients. He closed his office. Yet an online rating site gave him the "Patient's Choice Award" two years later, a "Compassionate Doctor's Recognition Award" three years later, and (my favorite) the "On Time Doctor's Award" *five years* after his office was closed.
- A dead plastic surgeon, who had given up his license ten years earlier, was still receiving positive ratings. In fact, two years after his death, an online rating site was still reporting five out of five stars for his practice. A comment left months after he died stated, "I am beyond happy with my results…turned out better than I could have ever hoped for…I highly recommend people looking for a cosmetic surgeon to go there." A rating submitted three years after he died claimed, "They make me feel like I'm their only patient…I'm going to tell everyone about them…I absolutely love this place."

Because of the online ratings boom, physicians have felt pressured to hire marketing experts or reputation management firms to monitor the rating sites. These management firms give physicians "a dedicated team who will work every day to provide relevant and interesting content for websites that will get your practice noticed." I frequently receive unsolicited emails from marketing management firms. A recent email blast from a marketing consulting firm promised they'd "boost your ratings this summer, optimize SEO, and bring patients flooding to your door."

A marketing firm actually put out bad reviews for plastic surgeons on the online rating sites and then sent emails to these offices offering to "fix" the bad reviews.

Marketing experts convince plastic surgeons these rating sites are important. This has led to some outrageous ratings site manipulation—even by some of the best surgeons. A well-respected plastic surgery group in Missouri lost a patient because of their relentless desire for testimonials and ratings. This patient came to see me after consulting with a physician in this group. She was offered a significant discount on the cost of her procedure. All she had to do is visit three internet rating sites and, using her real first name so they could identify her for the discount, post a positive review. They didn't want her to do this after the procedure; they asked that she do it before having the work done! While my patient felt this request was inappropriate, I'm sure many other patients felt this was a great way to save money.

Rating sites care only about advertising and increasing traffic to their sites, which is why they give lip service to the phrase "verified reviews." One such site promises 100 percent verified reviews and ratings, but the physician has to pay to be on this rating site. Another website has been accused of filtering positive reviews and will show them only if the physician pays to advertise with them. Even Angie's List advertises "Reviews You Can Trust," which seems to say that you can't trust the other rating sites.

Physicians are told they can leverage online reviews to build up their online reputation. Marketing firms promise they'll deemphasize negative reviews and highlight five-star reviews. Many sites even elevate promoted posts (fee-based content that generates revenue for the site) over organic reaches or unpaid posts. One online reputation manager recently sent out an email blast to notify plastic surgeons that their company would "automatically generate new reviews and push them out to the internet… and drown out the negative reviews." Another firm promised a "backdoor trick," which was a "legal and a perfectly ethical loophole" that promised first-page Google rankings and five-star positive patient reviews.

Automated review software tools may also be purchased by providers. The automated software sends an invitation to patients asking them to post a review, but it will also screen patients so that unhappy patients will not be asked to submit a review. It filters reviews, sending only positive ones to the provider's website, social media, or prominent third-party review sites. It scans the internet sites and selects which sites to send the patient reviews based on the need for more positive reviews on that site or simply the need for new reviews. It will even cut and paste reviews from one site to another and make minor changes in the wording so as to not damage SEO.

A website that went offline in 2016 called MyBadPlasticSurgery.com detailed the bad outcomes from one specific plastic surgeon. Some of the stories were gruesome. Worse, he's still in practice today. Below is the introduction to the site, which can still be found in the internet archives of the Wayback Machine:

> "Welcome to MyBadPlasticSurgery.com. The purpose of this site is to warn the public of not fully investigating your plastic surgeon. Unfortunately, this can become a daunting task due to the recent boom in SEO/internet marketing public relations firms. These firms make it their business to create fake pages and reviews of plastic surgeons. This can be extremely misleading to the unsuspecting public."

It's a shame this site doesn't exist anymore because it provided a useful service: a warning about the importance of researching your possible plastic surgeon by only using rating sites. I imagine it was pushed offline by marketing firms.

2,000 Followers

Social media is a visual tool that allows users to share content and information with the public via virtual communities and networks. That means you can put something out on a social media platform and billions of people can theoretically find and see it. Unfortunately, it also never goes away nor is erased. Social media platforms include Facebook (2.2 billion monthly active users), YouTube (1.9 billion), Instagram (1 billion), X (formerly Twitter, 556 million), and Snapchat (255 million). Social media does provide a better return on investment (ROI) than other marketing, including print and billboards.

It is important to state up front that I am biased against self-promotion on social media or even advertising. I did not even list in the "yellow pages" of a phone book back in the day. I just want prospective patients to be able to find me if they know my name. This has worked well for me, but I understand that it is not for everyone. Now people are impressed by someone's "followers" on social media, but the number of "followers" can be manipulated and even bought, similar to online rating sites. This has led to many physicians trying to "outdo" each other to attract, educate, and maintain their patient base with many attractive forms of entertainment. Sometimes this entertainment hovers between appropriate and inappropriate but almost always compromises the doctor/patient professional relationship. A good plastic surgeon's greatest concern should be for the patient and not what benefits, including financial, the surgeon will have with more "patients" or "followers."

Some patients, unfortunately, go to see a plastic surgeon because of their internet presence on social media. Board certification is more important than having 2,000 followers (many who have never met the professional) or 20,000 likes. But most important, the number of "followers" does not tell a potential patient the plastic surgeon's education, experience, skill, or results.

What is the bottom line? Be thorough in your research and remember that most people placing reviews on the internet have an agenda. Once bad plastic surgery happens, it's hard to rectify and you'll never have the body or face you had before.

Chapter 7

Patients Share Responsibility
–Part 2

-- -- -- -- -- --

I n Chapter 3, "Natural and Aesthetic Ideals," I introduced the concept of mathematical ratios to explain how beauty is defined. These mathematical ratios translate into proportional aesthetics—the placement of features that are pleasing to the eye.

In this chapter, a continuation of the idea that *patients share responsibility*, we'll explore the fourth of the reasons for bad plastic surgery I presented in Chapter 6: ignoring the big picture of your appearance, having skewed or unconventional aesthetics, or holding unrealistic expectations about what can be done can make a plastic surgeon's job much more difficult and can produce results that aren't aesthetic, mathematically proportional, and are, at times, strange or hideous.

Magnifying Mirrors

Mirrors with five- or ten-times magnification were meant to help the vision of the older eye. But over time, these mirrors have become staples in many women's homes, young and old. It's the unfettered use of these strong magnifiers that's causing women unnecessary consternation. Using these magnifying mirrors does two things: 1) they magnify the small problems, and 2) they eliminate seeing the big, overall picture of your appearance.

When you look at a magnifying mirror, you'll see things no one else sees. Every little pore will be magnified and every red area will seem like an infected boil. Anyone who looks at you won't see these things because they're standing at a distance from you. For some women, using a magnifying mirror becomes an obsession almost bordering on a disorder. Patients who stare at their image in the mirror for hours will suddenly see that one eye is smaller or lower, one eyebrow is higher, one nasal opening looks wider, more wrinkles are on the lower lip than the upper lip, and more wrinkles are around the right eye than the left eye.

I had a patient who wasn't able to tell me what was wrong with her face without reaching for the five-times magnifying mirror in the exam room. She was shocked when I told her that I couldn't appreciate the problem she was complaining about on her face. I'm sure that another surgeon "saw it" and "fixed it" for her, hopefully to her satisfaction. I had another patient grab a mirror to show me the lines that bothered her. Turns out, they were smile lines around her eyes that appeared when she fully smiled. These lines seemed more severe in the mirror but were very minimal and natural in real life.

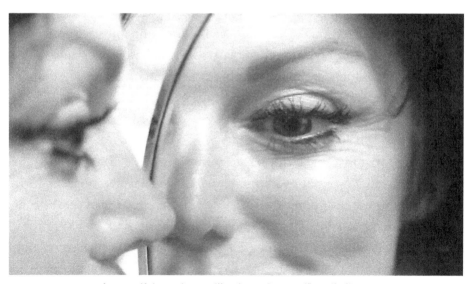

A magnifying mirror will enlarge "normal" smile lines
and make them look more severe.

Mirrors also only offer a two-dimensional view, which alters lines and shadows, making them appear abnormal. In a three-dimensional view, those same lines and shadows look appropriate. It's important to look at the overall picture and not become obsessed with the small things, because small things are even smaller in the big picture. I'm not advocating throwing these magnifying mirrors away, but I do ask that you use them prudently. If you look at yourself in a magnifier, also be sure to look at yourself in a full-length mirror—stand about six feet away—to see yourself as others see you.

Imposing Requests or Limits on Your Surgeon

Your surgeon should have the skill to offer what they think will give you the best result. However, sometimes patients impose requests, such as a desire for a specific procedure, that place restrictions on what the surgeon can do.

Patients call my office inquiring if I do Smart Lipo, the ThreadLift, or Gummy Bear implants. Others call asking if we have Juvéderm, Sculptra or Botox. Still others call asking if we perform fractional laser resurfacing, chemical peels, or dermabrasion. A patient once called requesting a "deep plane facelift that I saw on the internet."

Instead of choosing a plastic surgeon based on reputation, recommendations, or experience, these patients are choosing their surgeon based on whether or not they can perform their chosen procedure. These patients aren't looking for a critical evaluation by a physician. They've already chosen their procedure based on advertisements and the internet and apparently think that every outcome is the same no matter who performs the procedure. This couldn't be further from the truth.

When patients request a specific procedure, I usually answer that I do that procedure but only when it's indicated or necessary. I always ask them why they feel that procedure is appropriate for them since all techniques have advantages, disadvantages, and limitations. Most of the time, the patient doesn't know why they want it; they just do. I usually direct these patients to someone in town doing that specific procedure although I may also perform that requested procedure. They don't understand that who does the procedure is more important than the procedure itself.

As noted earlier in the book, some patients are adamant they don't want surgery, even minimally invasive surgery. This could be because they're scared or they believe the effects will be too obvious and that people will know they've had "work done." Such is often the case for the patients who request fat injections and want nothing else. To be clear, fat injections are amazing on the right face. But if the patient has very deflated, lax facial skin with poorly positioned supporting structures, so much fat has to be injected to fill the loose skin and improve the wrinkles that the patient's face will look "pillowy," without definition. In this case, a facelift and a small amount of filler over the cheekbone would give this patient the most natural result.

Other patients are okay with surgery but insist it must be minimally invasive. These patients believe that if less is done, the changes will be less obvious or noticeable to others. But more extensive surgery doesn't necessarily mean that the results are more noticeable. In fact, minimal surgery may be more noticeable because it hasn't fully corrected the deformity. For example, a mini tummy tuck will only address the fat and the loose skin below the belly button. If you needed a full tummy tuck but requested only a mini tummy tuck, you'll be left with bulging in the upper part of your abdominal wall because of loose, separated muscles and skin excess. Repositioning the support structures to their expected position and skin excision is better than just moving the skin over the top of a malpositioned support structure.

The familiar "tight" look many people associate with facelifts of old may happen during "skin-only" or "mini" facelifts. This appearance occurs when the skin is pulled over the sagging support structures of the face. The patient's face may look tighter, but it won't look younger or better. A full facelift will correct the underlying structures of the face and neck and drape the skin to give a natural rejuvenation. The outcome will appear more balanced since the crepe-like neck skin will be corrected as well. This correction doesn't occur during a skin-only facelift, leaving the patient with a tight face but a less-than-youthful neck. If you need a facelift, you need a facelift. Anything less (i.e., fat injections) won't give you facelift results.

Some patients insist that all they need is a "mini tuck." I think they ask for it because they don't want to feel bad that they need a full tummy tuck and will feel better thinking they only require a mini tuck. Other patients won't consider a full tummy tuck because of the longer recovery time and the longer scar that's created. It's best to follow your surgeon's recommendation of liposuction versus tummy tuck or mini versus full tummy tuck. The improved results will be worth it.

Liposuction is another procedure patients request to correct abdominal wall abnormalities, not really understanding who good candidates for this minimally invasive surgery are. Sometimes patients aged thirty to fifty undergo liposuction with good results, but liposuction alone is generally successful only in younger patients. The patients most likely seeking a major improvement in their abdominal wall are women who've had children and are left with loose skin, a lower abdominal protrusion, stretch marks, and a wide muscle separation. If only liposuction is performed, these patients will still be left with loose skin, a lower abdominal wall protrusion, stretch marks, and a wide muscle separation.

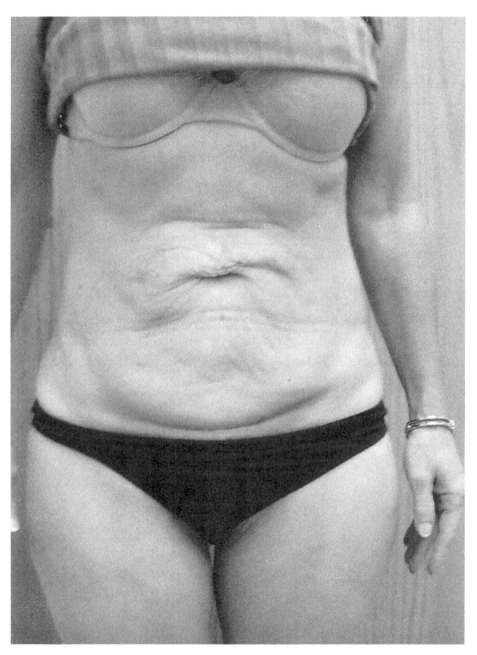

This patient would have received a much better result if a full tummy tuck was performed and not just the liposuction that she had one year earlier. She is still left with a separation of her abdominal muscles, loose skin, and stretch marks.

Only a full tummy tuck, which removes loose skin and stretch marks and tightens the muscle to correct the lower abdominal pooch, will provide the results these patients are seeking. The patient who insists on liposuction alone will be left with an unaesthetic result that may even be frightening to see when she wears a swimsuit.

Patients often request nasal surgery to be performed in a minimal way because they want to avoid the overcorrected surgery results from previous decades, including the overly scooped out nose (done when removing a bump) or the turned up nasal tip (which allows people to look up into the nose). If a surgeon performs a limited surgery as the patient requested, the patient likely will be very disappointed when the splint is removed on the first postoperative visit. Because of the limits imposed by the patient, the result may not be exactly what they'd envisioned. Surgeons can't read their patients' minds. This is why conversations about expectations are so important.

Ethnicity can be seen in the nose, and ethnic-erasing nasal surgery is frequently life altering. For some patients, years of prejudicial behavior and ill will toward them pushes them to erase their obvious ethnicity. Some patients, however, simply want to minimize, not eliminate, this feature. This minimization request can leave a surgeon perplexed because it may be difficult to achieve a look that's pleasing to the patient and also retains "enough" of their ethnicity. I experienced this firsthand with a patient who was born in India. On two different preoperative visits, we discussed the plans for her nose, and the agreed-upon result included some fairly significant changes. On the morning of surgery, she asked that I do less in order to maintain her ethnicity. We went ahead with the surgery, but I was left wondering how I was supposed to know what she considered ethnic enough. I did my best to meet her expectations by using a "less is more" approach, but she was somewhat unhappy that I hadn't made more changes to her nose.

Wanting Just a Little Bit More or a Little Bit Less

If a patient is unhappy with the results of a surgical procedure, their response is to want a little bit more added or a little bit more removed *right away*. The main problem with doing another procedure so soon is that the body doesn't respond well to multiple traumatic insults in a short time frame. The human body must go through different phases of healing before reaching a point where another procedure won't do more harm than good.

The *acute* phase of healing occurs two to three days after the initial injury. This phase is when bleeding, swelling, and bruising are at their worst. The *repair*, or *inflammatory*, phase starts at one week and lasts up to six weeks. During this phase, the tissues are inflamed and the body is laying down collagen to repair and strengthen the area of injury. The *remodeling* phase may last up to three months after the inflammatory phase, during which the tissue is strengthening and maturing. If the body is in the inflammatory phase of healing, adding another insult (e.g., surgery or injection) will drastically increase the inflammation and subsequently increase scarring at the site.

A new patient asked me to correct her upper eyelids after three rounds of surgery. Her surgeon had done a standard conservative upper lid skin removal initially. At her first postoperative visit, the patient complained that she could still "pull" the skin on her upper eyelid. The surgeon redid the surgery two weeks after the first (during the inflammatory phase) only to have the patient request a further resection of skin. One month later (and still in the inflammatory phase), and six weeks after the first surgery, the surgeon redid her upper lids and also "threw in" the lower lids because of her anger. Her result after multiple surgeries wasn't only aesthetically unnatural, but also left her unable to fully close her eyes. She couldn't protect both corneas from drying out at night, even when she taped her eyes shut. This was extremely painful for her throughout the night, limiting her ability to sleep and causing her further depression and distress.

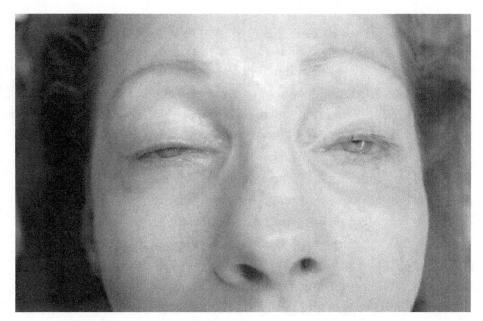

A patient who after her second eyelid surgery in three months could not close her eyes even at night and had to cover her eyes with her hands in the shower to prevent the water from hurting her corneas.

The phases of healing apply to all parts of the face and body, and operating again too soon will often cause more problems than it solves. Michael Jackson's nose illustrates what can happen when too many procedures are done too close together. The absolute worst result happened to a man after he had twelve surgeries on his nose. It had to be amputated because it was beyond repair.

Just going a little bigger with breast implants seems easy enough, but you always risk losing the implants to infection after secondary surgeries, especially if it's done too soon after a previous surgery. Secondary breast surgery is fraught with the complications of recurrent scarring and nerve injuries, including loss of nipple sensation and the need for even more surgery. A plastic surgeon I know believes in the concept of "one and done" and reports a zero percent revision rate on his breast augmentation patients. He firmly believes he only has one surgery to make the breasts perfect and won't do secondary revisions on his patients.

I've had patients request more skin removal after a tummy tuck. They'll sit down and then grab some extra skin of the lower abdominal wall and ask, "Why is this still here?" I have to point out to them that the extra skin is needed to allow them to stand upright and is no longer extra when the patient is standing. Further skin removal in this situation would be unwise. The patient would be unable to stand completely upright and sport a wide, stretched-out scar.

Telling a surgeon before liposuction, "When you feel that you are done suctioning, keep on going," isn't only dangerous, it's counterproductive to the desired outcome. And, honestly, over-suctioning during liposuction is one of the biggest contributors to bad plastic surgery. Liposuction is as much art as science. The surgeon must determine how much fat can be removed without extracting too much, which would leave the skin without its supporting foundation and result in loose, hanging skin or soft tissue deformities.

The body provides the definitive end point for suctioning an area. When liposuction begins, the first material that comes out is the yellow/white fat. However, after suctioning the same area for a while, the material coming out has more blood in it and the fat starts to thin. Soon after the thinning fat appears, suctioning should be stopped. If suctioning continues, the material removed becomes all blood and no fat. At this point, the surgeon is only traumatizing the tissues as most of the fat has already been removed. The instrument starts to rip and tear blood vessels, nerves, and lymphatic tissue. If the suction is performed closer to the skin and the cushioning fat is removed, the patient may be left with contour deformities and skin irregularities. It's best to let the surgeon determine when they're "done."

Lasers are another tool that can be overused. Frances learned this the hard way and presented with a waxy appearance due to the overuse of lasers. But using a laser is like driving a car. If you push a car to one hundred miles per hour, you're more likely to have a serious accident. If you push a laser to get a greater than 20 percent improvement, you're going to cause serious burn injuries to the skin.

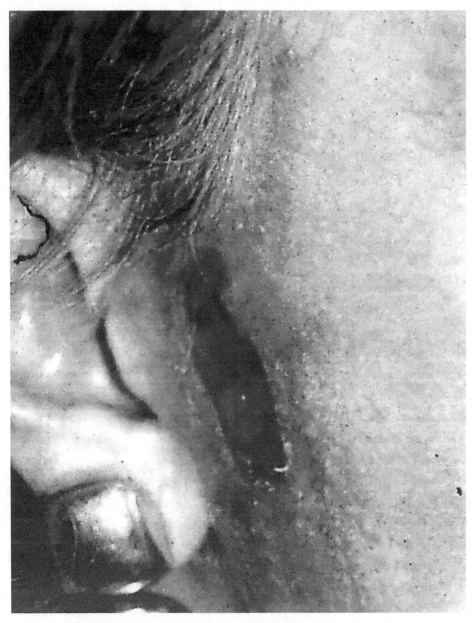

The patient sustained a laser burn to her right cheek trying to take
her skin tightening to a higher level.

Fillers and neuromodulators can often be overdone for the sake of "wanting a little bit more." I like to keep some motion in the muscles after a neuromodulator injection, but some patients want just a little more injected so that nothing moves in their forehead. A patient of mine came in religiously for cheek injections. She'd even ask to see the syringe after I finished to make sure I'd used it all during the injection session. After a number of sessions, I felt she was full enough based on her appearance and refused to inject her. She returned three months later, requesting more material to fill her cheeks. To my eye she was still filled enough and I passed on injecting her that day. She failed to show for her next visit.

About a year later, by chance we attended the same reception. My daughter spotted my former patient first. She asked me, "What's the matter with that lady's face over there?" I recognized my previous patient, and it was obvious she'd gone to someone else to get further injections. Her cheeks were so ballooned that even my young daughter appreciated just how bad she looked. I received an update about my former patient three years later from a current patient. She told me the woman had had even more filler and looked both hideous and hilarious. For this patient, always wanting *just a little bit more* ended up looking like bad plastic surgery. Sometimes, a little is good. Usually, a lot is not.

Supersize Me

I was surprised the first time a patient said, "Please supersize me," as if she were ordering fast food. She'd fallen for the idea that "big is good and more is better." This belief can be applied to the face, breast, buttocks, and genitalia and typically means as it sounds. In the animal world, well-endowed animals are more attractive to the opposite sex.

One such supersizing that's frequently seen in the animal kingdom involves the male ballooning out his cheeks to attract a female. Hollow cheeks are viewed as old and weak, whereas authority is associated with strong cheek structure. The partner with the stronger cheeks is said to control romance and marriage. Similarly, thin, small, and narrow lips generally define an unemotional, selfish, and miserly character whereas large, full, round lips ooze sensuality. A person with large lips is characterized as sensitive, caring, expressive, and somewhat hedonistic. Lip size and color may also be the first outward sign to stimulate attraction from another.

While the attraction of large breasts relates to increased breast size around menstrual cycles, pregnancy, and nursing, supersizing a breast destroys all the landmarks associated with a pleasing, beautiful breast. The implants are out of proportion to the chest and extend beyond the boundaries of the normal breast. This projection is unnatural compared to the diameter. The volume doesn't adhere to body proportions, and there's no increased lower fullness compared to an unexpected upper fullness of the breast. The implants appear to be two huge balloons or melons placed on a woman's chest. There's rarely separation between the breasts, which creates unnatural cleavage. The outward pressure of the implant on the soft tissue thins the breast tissue and skin causing unsightly wrinkling. Nothing is aesthetically pleasing about a supersized breast.

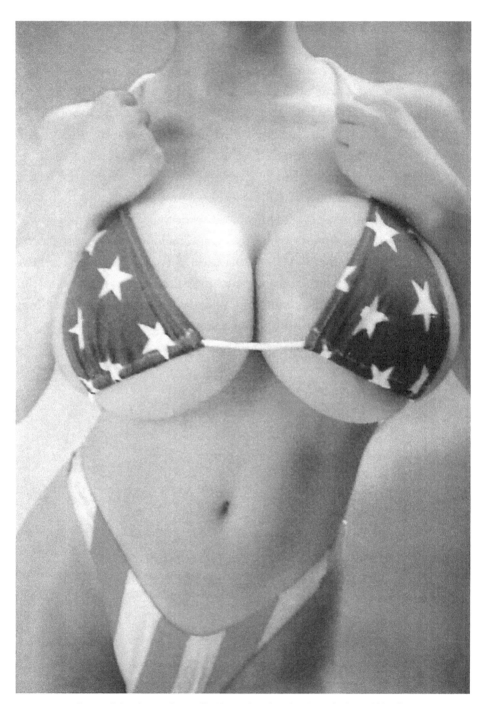

Supersizing is rarely aesthetic and makes buying clothes difficult.

There can be a lot of associated problems.

In the primate world, the buttocks are used for attracting the opposite sex. The female macaque monkey will swell her scarlet buttocks with blood when she's ready to mate. The male mandrill monkey has vibrant red buttocks that are displayed to the female as a secondary sexual characteristic. It isn't a stretch to suggest that the display of a round, female hemispheric buttock is used in humans as a sexual attraction. As with the breasts, increased roundness and size is associated with increased fertility, making the female attractive to the male. An erotic beauty is also associated with increased buttock size and fat content.

If big is good, bigger is better. This has led to a segment of supersized, bad plastic surgery buttocks. A buttock lift will tighten and raise the buttocks, but it adds little fullness. To increase the size of the buttocks and add fullness, silicone implants have been tried and have mostly failed due to a high complication rate, including infections and exposure of the implant. Fat injections add some fullness and roundness, but they're prone to poor viability because patients sit on them, which crushes the transferred fat prior to full revascularization.

Because of the problems and costs associated with buttock implants and fat grafting, nonqualified providers have taken to injecting buttocks with household items including caulk, beeswax, glue, nonmedical silicone, and wood-patching compounds. With these artificial fillers, buttocks can be overfilled but with horrible complications that result in bad plastic surgery.

Distinguished genitalia can be important in the primate world. The male vervet monkey possesses a pale blue scrotum and a red penis to attract females. Patients have also asked to "supersize" and distinguish their genitalia to increase their erotic beauty. They have been known to bring in artificial replicas of their favorite porn stars and ask to look like their idols. Some patients request "labial puff" injections, an attempt to fill out the deflated, aged labia. Labial aesthetic surgery typically involves matching the patient's labia to something they've seen in pornography, on a friend or partner, or a vaginal substitute. Prior to seeing these other labia examples, the patient probably didn't think their labia were abnormal. In fact, they may possess normal labia, but now that they've seen something different, they want *that* to be their normal. It should be noted that some extremely long or large labia can cause local problems of irritation and occasional infection and should be corrected. The number of patients seeking labial reduction surgery has increased significantly over the last few years.

One prospective male patient came to me years ago with a penile substitute requesting a similar one himself because "My partner enjoys this more than mine." Penile implants and fat grafting to increase the girth of the penis have an exceedingly high complication rate. Penile implants can become infected which has led to amputation of the penis. Fat grafting of the penis shaft has resulted in irregularities because the fat is placed superficially and may disturb sensation and the ability to have an erection. Silicone injections into the penis have led to death.

Some patients go to these supersizing extremes to irk a previous partner. This is called "revenge plastic surgery" and affects both sexes, although it tends more to be a woman getting back at a straying husband. They want the ex-partner jealous about what they no longer can have. The movie *First Wives Club* illustrated this concept when one jilted wife had her lips supersized after her husband left her. Large, full lips, being a hallmark of erotic beauty, are a common revenge plastic surgery favorite. I've injected the cheeks of two women who went through expensive, nasty divorce proceedings. They were attempting to restore a fuller, more youthful face as well as give themselves a more authoritative appearance as they reentered the dating circuit.

Supersized breast augmentation is also used as revenge plastic surgery. It's pretty obvious how this is getting back at a former partner. Larger breasts may have been something the ex-partner had requested. Obtaining them after the relationship is over is a way for a woman to show her ex that she has something he'll never enjoy. Once I was preparing a patient for breast enlargement surgery and asked if her husband, whom I'd met at her preoperative consultations, was there for me to talk to after the surgery. She giggled and responded, "He'll never see these, although he paid for them. He's getting divorce papers served at his office while I'm in surgery." Ouch! The perfect revenge is completed.

Men use revenge plastic surgery less, but will typically address love handles, the eyes, or the neck after a relationship ends. Occasionally, penile enhancements are done as well.

The Appeal of "Plastic" Hollywood

Hollywood doesn't allow its stars to age. By the time stars reach age 34, their salaries have significantly dropped if they can find work at all. Most stars feel that they have to make the most of what they've got while they've got it. Audrey Munson may have been the first actress to feel this isolation as she aged.[13] She was known as the "American Venus" and was cast as a sculptor's model in the 1915 movie *Inspiration*. In this role, she was the first actress ever to be filmed fully nude in a nonpornographic movie production. Early in her career, she was chosen as the model for many statues in New York City. She subsequently went on to become what we'd consider today a supermodel. Sadly, as she aged, she faded into the unknown. At thirty, a judge committed her to a psychiatric facility, where she remained until her death sixty years later.

> *Worldly fame is but a breath of wind that blows now this way and now that, and changes name as it changes direction." (Dante Alighieri, 1265–1321)*

Hollywood is a town where looks are everything. But human beings age and actors have to cope with this process. Some have decided to thwart the aging process. This list may include Cindy Crawford, Sally Field, Marie Osmond, and Raquel Welch. When looking at their photographs, it's hard to tell which photos are from the past and which are more recent. I believe these celebrities are having small procedures done to keep them looking fresh-faced. Their plastic surgeons are using a light touch to restore these star's faces as they age without altering their features in a way that would give them a different or unnatural look.

If there's anything that's constant in Hollywood, it's change. Actors can rise quickly and fall even quicker. To stay in the spotlight and pertinent, actors need to be able to reinvent themselves, accept different roles, and adopt a new look. Needing to have this "chameleon-like" ability is understood even by the young actors just starting their careers. It's possible that this adaptability has gone a little too far, because today's older actors, to attract more attention, are tending toward exaggerating their looks with artificial youthful beauty rather than a more naturally aged look. These unnatural changes can include large, pouty lips, overfilled high cheekbones that cause the eyes to appear small and sunken, and large, round buttocks. Of course, no change would be complete without breast implants. Large, bouncy breasts are almost a necessity now if only to fill out a bikini top in case their picture ends up on the front page of a tabloid magazine. Men aren't immune to these changes as a sculpted chin and jawline, as well as defined abdominal muscles, are sometimes taken to the extreme.

Because Hollywood celebrities are shattering traditional body and aesthetic standards, they're broadening what now is acceptable in society. These strained ideals also mean hearing people say, as these transformed actors walk the red carpet, "That doesn't look like them at all!" Much of Hollywood is taking good plastic surgery to the extreme, which contributes to some of the plastic surgery nightmares you see in the red-carpet parade. But celebrities have a lot of money. They can go to the best plastic surgeons and pay exorbitant sums to remake their faces and bodies. Are older actors helping or hurting their careers with extreme, unnatural plastic surgery? Yes, they look different, but do they look better?

And just because celebrities can afford to hire the best and most expensive plastic surgeons, does this mean that their distorted, unnatural appearances are the way plastic surgery *should* look? After all, a trend begins after many people do the same thing. Is this what we should all desire?

Some people feel their body doesn't reflect who they are as a person and it's their prerogative if they want to change it. But when people try to look like a celebrity, they're often attempting to erase their own identity and mimic the celebrity's identity. While they might come close to looking like someone else, to be an exact match is extremely difficult due to the placement of individual bone structures and facial proportions. That doesn't mean people won't try, and over-the-top procedures frequently are employed when copying celebrity faces.

Celebrities aren't the only things people copy. A woman reportedly spent nearly one hundred thousand dollars to look like a blow-up sex doll. Other women have tried to look like a Barbie doll, which represents the ultimate in fake looks. Even men get into the act as they try to look like a Ken doll.

Perhaps the most perplexing are the people who undergo plastic surgery to look like an animal, a reptile, or a mythical creature. Examples include Jocelyn Wildenstein's feline characteristics, Dennis Avner's tiger features, Erik Sprague's lizard looks, and María José Cristerna's vampire warrior.

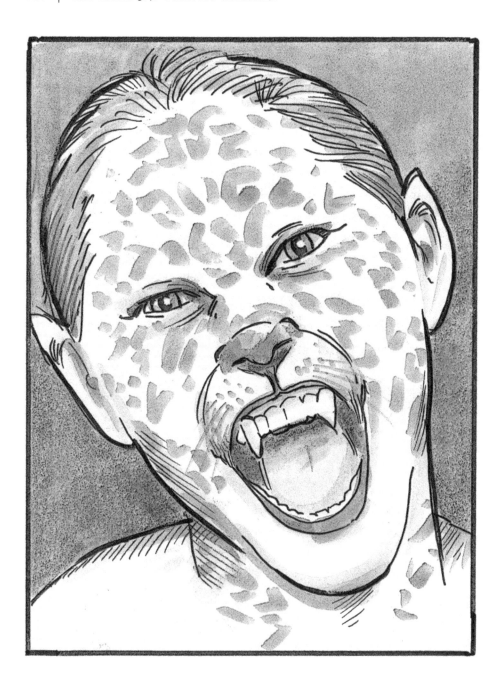

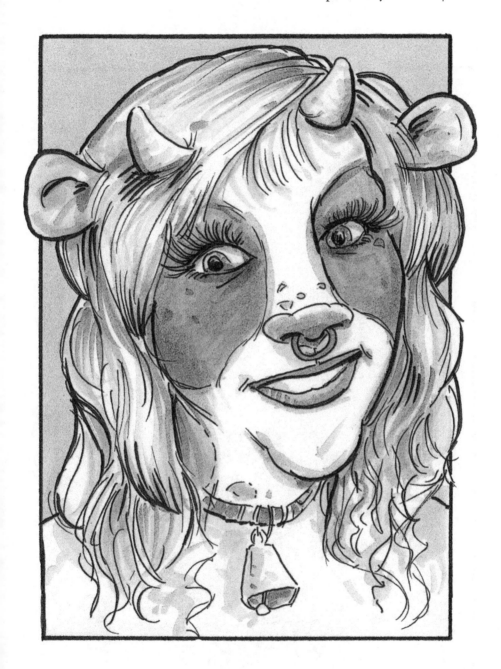

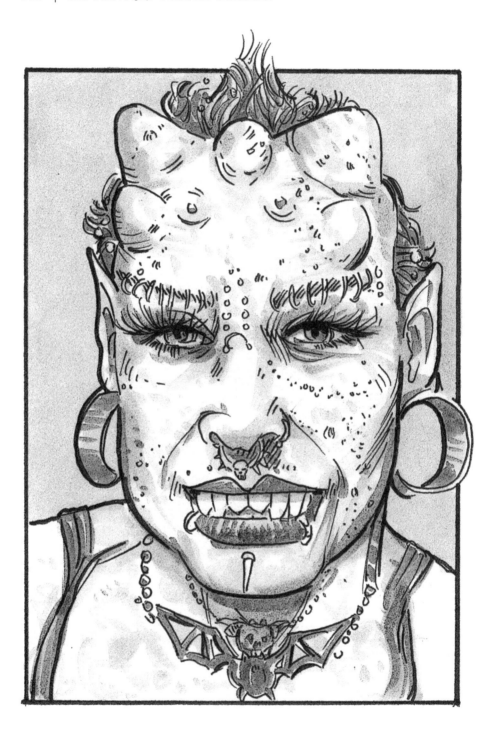

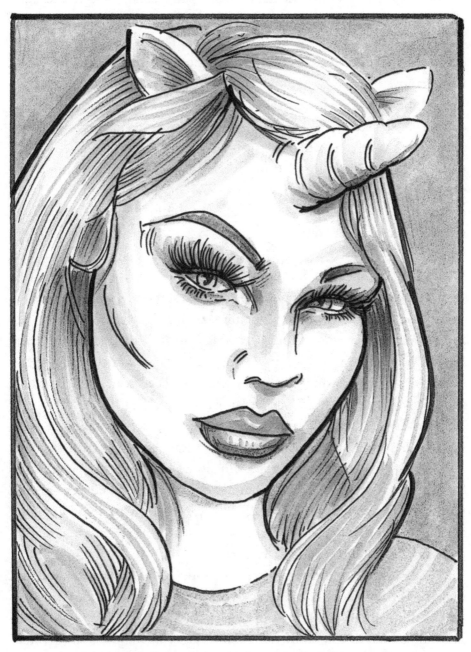

Some people try to mimic animals and duplicate the animal's
outward appearance onto themselves.

Unfortunately, these patients have lost their human looks in exchange for being different enough to warrant stares and gasps. A psychologist explained to me that they adopt these inhuman looks through plastic surgery to mask inner problems. I always wonder if this treatment makes them happy.

On the other hand, the plastic surgery they've had done, while difficult for most to look at, actually suggests skilled surgeons may have been at work. It's hard to create defects that plastic surgeons have been taught to correct, such as a feline cleft lip. It takes finesse to create bumps when plastic surgeons are often tasked with removing lumps and bumps. The outcome that these people wanted makes it a bit harder to see the artistry in the plastic surgeon's result.

Expecting Scar-Less Surgery

Any type of surgery creates scars. Plastic surgery is no exception. A good plastic surgeon will always emphasize that scarring will occur after surgery and will vary in visibility according to how the individual heals. A good way to know how a scar will look can be based on a previous scar. Aaron, mentioned earlier, was upset with his facial scars. Yet, he had a wide, raised scar after his appendectomy thirty years earlier.

Scars can be barely perceptible or can be raised, red, and wide. Any time the skin is cut, the patient is left with a scar. An incision will result in a good scar or a bad scar, but there will always be a scar. The potential of bad scarring is why some patients prefer noninvasive procedures—there's no cutting of the skin, hence no scar. You can't cut the skin and not leave a scar. Patients during consultations will exclaim, "There will be a scar?! I thought plastic surgeons didn't leave scars!"

Plastic surgeons do employ special considerations to decrease scarring, though. The first tactic is orienting the scar so that it lies within a natural fold of the body or along lines of relaxation. Lines of relaxation tend to run horizontally in the body but more vertical in the face. An example is the natural fold under each breast. An incision in this area isn't visible when looking straight on at the breast. It's only seen if the breast is lifted up. In the face, the natural fold from the nose to the corner of the mouth is often used when closing skin cancer excision defects since the fold hides the incision. If you look into a mirror and then smile, you'll see the animation lines on your face where an incision could be hidden. If an incision goes across these lines, the natural line is disrupted and the scar will tend to pull apart.

The length of the scar depends on the amount of skin removed. The scar will be approximately three times longer than the skin excision is wide. The length that adequately closes an incision also produces the most aesthetically pleasing scar. This technique is necessary to reduce the skin redundancies (sometimes called "dog ears") on either end of the incision. Patients are often flabbergasted by how long the scar is after tummy-tuck surgery because they can't always appreciate how much excess skin they have. If eight inches of skin is being removed from the lower abdomen during a tummy tuck, then the incision needs to be at least 24 inches long…over two feet in length. But it's always better to have an attractive longer scar than a short, unsightly scar.

The width of the scar depends on the amount of tension it must endure. Placing deep stitches can limit the width of a scar by better distributing the tension on the skin closure. In addition, putting in many stitches when closing an incision aids in relieving tension. This works because the more stitches placed, the less pull that's exerted on each stitch, decreasing the chance of the skin pulling. It's believed that decreasing the tension on a skin closure reduces scar formation by 90 percent.

Breast surgery presents a particular problem. Breasts can be the center of attention, and scars may distract from the aesthetics of soft and smooth breasts. In fact, breast scars tend to be wide because the breast implants create tension on the closures due to their increased volume. Breast reduction surgery can also have this issue despite reducing the volume of the breast. Since skin is removed and the breast skin is tightly pulled back together, the tension created may cause the scars to widen. Incisions around the darkened area of the nipple may leave a white scar, which can be noticeable due to the abrupt color change between the darkened areola and the lighter skin. In fact, The Doctors' Company, an insurance carrier for physicians, reported breast scars as one of the most common filings against plastic surgeons. A prominent plastic surgeon in Atlanta coined the term "Scar Wars" as surgeons attempt to change breast reduction and breast lift patterns to limit the extent of the scars.

To compound the scarring conundrum, different areas of the body can scar in distinctive ways. Eyelid scars tend to be fine in appearance because the skin there is very thin. Back scars are almost always wide because the skin is thicker. Plastic surgeons do everything they can to limit the scarring, but the way a scar heals is up to the patient. Topical treatments may help somewhat (steroids, silicone gel, onion extract, retinols, massage, etc.), but some patients just scar badly. Two breast reduction patients of mine had surgery on the same day using the same technique and closure of the incision. One patient's scar was a fine white line. The other patient's scar was wide and red because she had fair skin, red hair, and freckles.

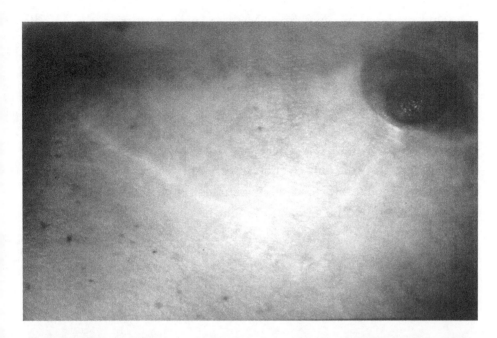

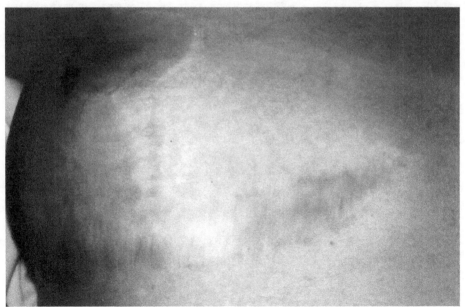

These two breast reductions were performed on the same day. One patient healed with a fine white line scar and the other patient's scar was wide and red although the breast reduction technique was the same.

Some darker skin types from Mediterranean countries, the Middle East, Central and South America, South Asia, Africa, and the Caribbean run the risk of developing keloid scars. Keloid scars are raised and painful while healing and extend beyond the initial injury drawing in the surrounding normal tissue.

Almost anyone can form a keloid on the chest even after minimal excisions. I've seen probably a half-dozen patients who had small moles removed from this area only to end up with much larger keloid scars. One patient had a small mole removed by a surgeon but ended up with a small keloid after healing. The surgeon thought he could remedy the situation if he excised the keloid. The patient ended up with a much larger keloid. The surgeon then attempted a fix by extending the incision and changing the direction of parts of the scar to "relax the tension," only to leave the patient with a scar nearly ten times the size of the original mole.

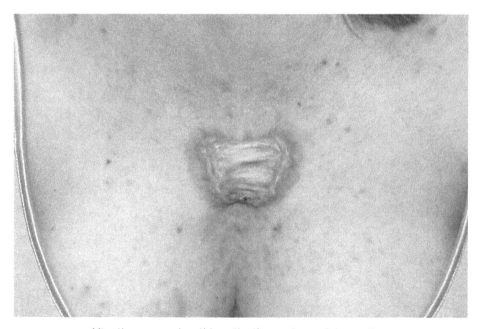

After three surgeries, this patient's scar is much larger than
the mole that was initially removed.

Another patient had heart surgery as a child only to have a large keloid develop in the upper part of the chest incision. It couldn't have developed in a worse place for a young lady, as it was visible in almost any shirt or blouse that she wore.

Most scars on the body tend to be less important because clothes usually cover them, as with a patient who'd developed keloid scars where every stretch mark appeared during her pregnancy. Marilyn Monroe's gallbladder removal scar is a classic bad scar, but it was usually covered by her clothes. Her scar seemed more of an issue for others, for she readily showed it in the partially clothed photo shoots she did later in life.

Fear of Missing Out (FOMO)

Our electronics-dependent society makes FOMO a common concern. FOMO is the apprehension that you may not be having the same rewarding experiences that others are having. If your friend gets the newest phone, then you need it also or you'll be missing out on the newest features. Unfortunately, FOMO drives a lot of decisions made by patients as well as providers. These decisions tend to involve the newest, latest, and greatest—but not always. Sometimes a decision is made simply to have or do what others have done or did.

One day, a patient called the office complaining that her skin care regimen didn't include Vitamin C. All her friends were using this "special" Vitamin C on their skin. When we informed her that one of the products she was using contained a more stable Vitamin C as well as other antioxidants, she still wanted the same name brand product her friends were using. She left the care of our office, probably going to her friend's skin care provider. Another patient called to ask why she wasn't using Retin A like her sister in California. Her sister said her skin was always red and flaking off because of the Retin A. It took some time for our patient to understand that she was using retinol mixed with both anti-inflammatories and antioxidants to utilize the effects of Vitamin A to the deeper skin cells while limiting the drying effect and injury to her skin surface that Retin A alone would have caused.

After seven years of successful results with one neuromodulator, a patient requested that we switch to the neuromodulator her daughter was receiving because it was "new and better." After one injection session, we switched back to the original neuromodulator we'd successfully used in her for years.

A potential breast augmentation patient wanted the same implants her friend had obtained from another plastic surgeon a few months before. The implants she wanted were inappropriate for her in many ways, including size, where they were placed, and the width of the implant. According to my evaluation, the patient needed smaller, less projecting, and wider implants under her muscle because of her chest anatomy. She had her implant wishes fulfilled by the other plastic surgeon but returned to my office three months later with tear-filled eyes. After allowing for complete healing, I replaced her original implants with the smaller and wider implants with excellent, natural-appearing results.

FOMO applies to all aesthetic technologies including lasers, ultrasound, skin tighteners, and fat removal. Just because someone you know had the procedure done doesn't make it the right one for you. Aesthetic treatments need to be individualized so patients obtain the best results. Don't let FOMO drive your aesthetic decisions.

Chapter 8
Men Are Different

- - - - - - - - - - - -

Women are overly hard on themselves when they look in the mirror, seeing issues and being hypercritical of their perceived flaws and imperfections. Most men, however, tend to see their looks quite differently. A friend of mine explained that when he looks at his reflection, he sees an authoritative face, strong arms, huge chest muscles, six-pack abs, and thick, muscular thighs. The reality is nothing like this vision. His face is deflated, his chest has developed man boobs, and its former girth has slipped down to his expanded waistline so much that his belly hangs over his belt, and his thighs could only be described as fat. Because of their adherence to this visual illusion, men frequently wait until late in the aging process before seeking plastic surgery remedies.

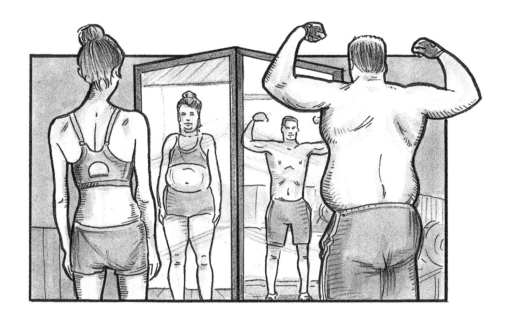

The unfortunate perception is that men look wiser and more distinguished as they age. This is truly regrettable because, when they're young, men rarely take the necessary precautions to reduce and slow the appearance of aging, including applying sunblock on their faces or wearing a hat. So, when a man does go to a plastic surgeon, he really needs intervention.

In the past, it was uncommon for men to have plastic surgery. Today, men now comprise approximately 20 percent of patients in many plastic surgeons' practices. The number of men undergoing cosmetic procedures is up 29 percent over the last ten years according to recent data from American Society of Plastic Surgery.[14] Terms specific to male procedures have been coined: Bro-tox and the Daddy Do-Over. Workplace pressure to look younger has increased since looking "aged" can damage job search activities. Then there are men who just want to look better.

By the time men get to a plastic surgeon, they're typically impatient and want a quick fix. Thus, men are less likely to do maintenance procedures such as fillers, neuromodulators, etc. and more likely to seek surgical corrections. But these corrections may pack more of a punch than men expect…or want.

Women frequently change their appearance through their makeup, hair, and clothes. Men, however, are less inclined to make even small changes and are less comfortable with *any* change in their appearance. Many men style their hair the same way for years—even when it's out of fashion—and insist on wearing that old, ratty T-shirt from a concert they attended twenty years earlier because "it still fits." Even minor changes appear major to someone who hasn't changed the way they look in years. Men would prefer to look five years better rather than fifteen years younger. In fact, looking too much better or too different can be disconcerting for some men. The bottom line is men don't always tolerate change well.

This intolerance of change is why men report being less happy with their plastic surgery results than women—as much as three times less happy regardless of the procedure performed. And some men are harder to please than most. The SIMON Syndrome (Single and Immature Male who is Overly expectant and Narcissistic) describes male cosmetic patients who are nearly impossible to satisfy even when they obtain a fabulous result.[15] These potentially problematic patients also often suffer from high anxiety and depression.

Dissatisfaction isn't relegated only to SIMON Syndrome sufferers. As a student of plastic surgery, I was taught to "rarely operate on a man's midline structure because men are never happy with it either before or after surgery." A surgeon I know operated on a man's nose. When the splint was removed, the surgeon thought that he'd "hit a home run because the result was superb." But the patient hated it. He became despondent over the surgery and began threatening the surgeon. For years, the patient told everyone how horrible the surgeon was and posted frequently on the online evaluation and rating sites. From all independent observers, he looked much better and had a more aesthetically pleasing nose to match his face. Yet he remained very unhappy.

One reason for male dissatisfaction and unhappiness with surgical results lies in the procedures themselves. Men want minor changes, yet many procedures are designed for women who can tolerate greater transformations. These procedures include brow lifts, eyelid surgery, and facelifts. Under the knife of a less skilled surgeon, men can end up with a too-high brow lift, beady eyes after eyelid surgery, and flat facial features and misaligned beard follicles after classical facelift procedures. All these things happened to my patient Aaron. His eyebrows were too elevated, his eyes were too squinty, his nose was too defined, and his skin was pulled too tight, which flattened his cheeks and brought his beard into his ear canal and behind his ears. An experienced plastic surgeon will adapt these typically female procedures so improvements are appreciated and extreme changes to male facial structures are avoided.

Finally, sometimes what appears to be bad plastic surgery is simply the path to a new and different life. Over the course of several years, Bruce Jenner, a male Olympic decathlon gold medal winner in the 1976 Olympics in Montreal, Canada, had numerous facial procedures performed that landed him on lists of celebrities who'd had bad plastic surgery. Those surgeries appeared to change his eyes, face, and nose, and reduce the prominent cartilage in his neck. Many critics commented how the procedures made him look feminine, which seemed to highlight the difficulties of performing aesthetic surgery designed for women on men.

In the spring of 2015, he underwent a final surgery that was reported to include a brow lift, reduction of his jawline, and augmentation of the cheeks, lips, and breasts. After ten hours, he emerged as Caitlyn Jenner. Gone were the heavy, low eyebrows on a prominent boney brow, the defined cheeks with lower cheek hollows, and the strong, established jawline and chin. The most recent surgery removed or softened his remaining male features and established feminine qualities to "his" face and chest. Add long dark hair and good makeup and Caitlyn Jenner is an attractive female who looks nothing like her age.

As Caitlyn, the years of surgeries finally made sense. Bruce Jenner was no longer seen as a victim of bad plastic surgery. The world could see that she was the culmination of a desire to reflect on the outside what was felt on the inside. What was initially considered bad surgery is now seen as appropriate and well done.

I have four thoughts I'd like men to consider:

1. Don't be fooled by what you see in the mirror. Try to see yourself as others see you.
2. Take care of your skin! Sunscreen, sunglasses, and hats are your best friends in the sun, wind, and snow.
3. Consider less-invasive treatments before jumping to plastic surgery. You'll be surprised how they can improve your looks in minimal ways that as a male you will appreciate.
4. When you're ready for plastic surgery, enlist the services of an experienced, board-certified plastic surgeon who will listen to your concerns and provide the result you desire.

Chapter 9
Body Image and the Mind

- - - - - - - - - - - -

P lastic surgery is designed to "repair and make whole that which is lost." It involves operations that change a person's appearance, which occasionally can have psychological implications.

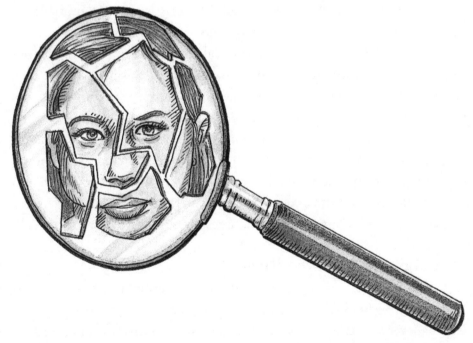

The effects of plastic surgery can be very beneficial, even life-changing. However it can also have negative effects because it results in an altered body perception. Body image is a dynamic and changing psychological progression. Some of these changes are positive, leading to enhanced self-esteem and greater joy in life. A young female shows improved self-esteem, confidence, and increased feelings of femininity after breast augmentation. But others are negative, causing emotional distress that leaves the person bereft and unhappy. A facelift may restore a youthful look, but it does not always improve the patient's self-esteem. Older patients, and especially men, may not tolerate body image changes as well as younger patients, and in some instances, the dramatic change after a facelift can cause the patient to become depressed and isolated.

During an initial evaluation, the plastic surgeon will supply information and answer the patient's questions. The surgeon should also assess the patient both physically and psychologically. This initial evaluation may be more important than the surgery itself. The plastic surgeon must determine if they can help the patient look better and, more importantly, feel better about themselves after the surgical intervention. An experienced surgeon will determine if the patient's concern is legitimate or are they obsessed with a negligible or even nonexistent "physical deformity." I was taught, "If I can't see it, I can't fix it."

When a surgeon identifies someone who has unrealistic expectations, expects perfection, or places too much importance on change, they should recommend psychiatric evaluation as a substitute for surgery. It can also be a preliminary step to prepare the patient for surgery. Plastic surgery may not be the best option and sometimes should not be performed at all.

That Can't Be Me in the Mirror!!!

Many of the patients I see tell me, "Overnight, everything has changed!" They're distraught and almost embarrassed because they didn't see what everyone else saw. Psychiatrists explain that this is a common phenomenon and it occurs in both men and women. We are conditioned to see ourselves as we did in our twenties or thirties. Since we don't see what everyone else sees, we don't appreciate the changes that have occurred. Then one day, usually after seeing a less than flattering image, reality sets in. With the next glance in a mirror, they see an old person looking back. It's not uncommon for patients to say, "Suddenly I look like my mom."

A patient once told me that this experience felt like "a reverse Dorian Gray moment." In the book *The Picture of Dorian Gray*, Dorian sells his soul so that a painted portrait of him will age but he'll remain youthful. As my patient suggested, she was aging, but her reflection in the mirror remained unchanged. She felt that she looked much younger and better than she really did.

What is the result of this delusion? Because of this phenomenon, patients have underappreciated the importance of prevention with lesser interventions. In youth, skin is well hydrated with great elasticity and without wrinkles. Thirty years of sun protection and good skin care, starting at age twenty years of age, *prevents* most signs of aging. *Correcting* skin laxity and wrinkles, after twenty-five years of little preventive care, becomes an uphill battle.

At eighteen years old, the skin is firm, plump, and radiant. It needs only protection from the sun. After twenty-five years, the skin needs to maintain hydration and protection (antioxidants and sunscreen). After forty-five years of environmental exposure, the skin needs repair using retinol and protection with antioxidants and sunscreen. Although it is never too late to start good skin care, it is best to start before aging is advanced. Dark spots, fine lines, and poor skin tone have created a great money-making opportunity for the beauty industry. It is very important for people to understand that it is going to take time, money, and a dedication to a skin care regimen if they are to see any improvement in the physical signs of aging. It is very difficult to reverse damaged skin; however, with appropriate skin care products, it can be accomplished or at least the damage can be slowed.

A more systematic approach may be needed to correct the damage from years of neglect. At this point, skin care alone won't remove wrinkles, sun damage, or improve skin laxity, and additional therapies may be necessary. Laser therapies at forty years old will help stimulate more collagen. Lasers or peels can remove dead skin cells, allowing new, healthy skin cells to emerge. When patients are older, age 50 and up, the skin cells don't function as efficiently and consequently produce less collagen. More aggressive laser treatments at age sixty will be needed to stimulate the same amount of collagen as less-invasive laser treatments would have done at age forty. The key to any preventive therapy is consistency. Prescription medications such as insulin and blood pressure medication don't work well if taken only half the time, and similarly, skin care products or laser therapies do little if used inconsistently.

Procedures done on youthful skin also last longer. Minor, less aggressive surgical procedures (such as neck liposuction) are more successful since younger skin is more elastic and will snap back in place after surgery. Removing a small amount of skin over the youthful, deep structures will rejuvenate a forty-year-old face without resulting in a "done" or "pulled "look as it would in an older patient with lax support and unhealthy, thin skin. When small, subtle changes are made, a youthful appearance continues. If you know someone who doesn't seem to age, it is probably because they continue with subtle treatments and consistent care of their skin.

Since more extensive, structural intervention needs to be done on an older person, the changes will be more obvious. Pulling on thin, inelastic skin often produces unsightly sweeps of the existing skin and wrinkles. Tension makes surgery look unnatural. Also, pulling on inelastic skin causes early relaxation, and the procedure's improvements are only short lived. Results on aged skin may last only three to five years; yet younger patients may see the improvements for decades.

Appropriate rejuvenation of the face is a continuance. Don't be shocked by your own "reverse Dorian Gray moment." Waiting until you feel desperate to have something done means undergoing more invasive treatments to achieve only moderate results. Deeper chemical peels, more painful laser therapies, or extreme surgery will be required to correct issues that could have been addressed earlier in a less-invasive way by years of good skin care, enhancing laser therapies, and appropriately early surgical interventions. Years of neglect will require more severe and exaggerated treatments that may result in unattractive, bad results.

Because the "Reverse Dorian Gray" phenomenon causes people to think they look younger and better than they actually do, it may also interfere with the perceived success of rejuvenation surgery.

An aged woman requesting eyelid and facelift surgery wanted to look "freshened up." Her family and friends constantly told her she looked tired and old. After her surgery, everyone told her how wonderful and alert she appeared and that she looked twenty years younger. Her husband and family were ecstatic, and yet she seemed disappointed. When I asked her about this, she confided in me that she saw no real improvements and that she felt she looked the same as she did before her surgery. We sat down together and looked over her preoperative and postoperative photographs, side by side. She confessed that she never realized she looked as aged as she did before surgery. *She WANTED to see the younger person she saw in the mirror and such was her perception.* She always saw the reflection in her mirror as a person who was 20 years younger and found it hard to believe the preoperative photos were really of her. Unfortunately, the results of the rejuvenation surgery, a good result by all standards, left her feeling confused and disappointed.

Making Changes for Changes' Sake

Some people deal with change better than others. For the majority of people, change is welcomed as a way to look and feel better. Some are comfortable with the natural appearance of aging, yet others do not feel that their aging face matches how they feel inside. Therefore, many explore the possibility of change through plastic surgery as a way to *look on the outside the way they feel on the inside.*

Women are accustomed to changing and enhancing their looks. They wear makeup, change hair color, and consistently update their style with wardrobe changes. They are critical of themselves but are not obsessed. These women will happily undergo surgery to reverse the signs of aging. They understand that a facelift does not remove every wrinkle or lift every part of the aging face. They realize regular visits to their plastic surgeon will maintain and enhance their improvements. They spend the time and money necessary to keep themselves looking as good as possible. We have all seen this attractive, put-together woman at the airport, businesses, and restaurants. She has glowing skin, appears younger than her age, and displays self-confidence.

Some women can have a surprising reaction to the process of aging and change. They may be open to drastic changes that result in a more plastic appearance. They are accustomed to seeing extreme surgical results on the streets of New York and Hollywood, as well as on television or Instagram. Their perception of beauty may be altered because they are more accustomed to seeing extreme and even "bad plastic surgery." You may see these deeply tanned women looking "different" and outdated. They may have a facelift that is pulled too tight, which may make them appear less attractive as they walk around in a track suit at the airport or mall.

Men don't always embrace change well. They don't feel the need to make changes to their appearance or their wardrobe. They have the same hairstyle their entire life and typically always do the same things. This is why they have deserved a chapter on their own.

The Revolving Door of Plastic Surgery

And then there are the people who see change as a way to reinvent themselves repeatedly. They may undergo the same procedure multiple times to gain a bigger "wow factor." They may attempt diverse procedures during one surgical event to completely modify their face and body. It's quite possible these surgical alterations are driven by insecurity and the desire to feel an immediate sense of gratification and happiness. Sadly, some of these people lose sight of how things may affect them long-term and undergo surgery impulsively because they want immediate change.

Celebrities are probably the worst offenders of revolving-door plastic surgery.

- A reality star had undergone twelve aesthetic procedures before she was twenty-four! The procedures included a brow lift, ear pinning, chin reduction, nose revision, and breast implants. Three years later, she underwent breast reduction surgery.

- A *Playboy* model credits her multiple breast surgeries for her ongoing success—at 22!
- An actress who played a television lifeguard had multiple breast surgeries to make her breasts bigger, then smaller, then bigger again.

These patients are hooked on change. They crave being noticed and are seeking compliments and praise for the "new addition." Sometimes this need for change becomes an addiction and leads to extreme or bad plastic surgery, but change makes them feel happy and—almost like a heroin addict—they constantly search for that "high" again. Some lose sight of how things may affect them long-term and undergo surgery impulsively because they want immediate change.

Plastic Surgery at Young Ages

All humans have insecurities, and for young people, their appearance creates the most anxiety and insecurity. According to a number of psychiatrists I know, having plastic surgery done at a young age can be the catalyst for an addiction to change. To avoid this, the process must be managed well by the surgeon and the parents. The key is to stifle the belief that plastic surgery is the answer to every physical issue and focus instead on accepting that imperfection is part of life.

A 22-year-old woman came to me asking for a *third* breast augmentation surgery because she wanted to go bigger. Her breasts were already out of proportion to the rest of her 128-pound frame after her first two surgeries. Because I discourage breast augmentation surgery until the patient is at least 20 years old, she had had her first two surgeries done by another surgeon. I passed on her third surgery, but I'm sure she found someone else to cater to her need for change. While I hope I'm wrong, I believe she'll continue on this path until a complication necessitates the removal of her implants. Should that happen, she'll be devastated.

What Drives Decisions

I've sought psychiatrists to help with the appropriate treatment when patients make inappropriate requests. A good working relationship with several psychiatrists has been invaluable in treating this type of patient.

For example, during a breast augmentation consultation years ago, I recommended an implant size to match her body, but she chose one of the smallest implants available. As an office, we spend a lot of time helping a patient choose the appropriate implant size based upon breast measurements, body type and frame, and trying to achieve a balanced appearance. Six weeks after the first surgery, after the swelling had resolved, she requested a larger implant. We encouraged her to choose the size we recommended. After waiting for full healing, the implants were exchanged for the size she requested, which was still less than the size we recommended. At first, she thought they were perfect. But once the swelling resolved, she wanted a larger size.

After a long discussion, I reluctantly performed the third surgery. Before entering her exam room four months after the third surgery, my nurse motioned me off to the side to say, "You won't believe this. She wants to be bigger *again*." In that moment, I realized she had an issue that was beyond my scope of understanding. I told her I'd perform one more surgery for her without charge if she'd submit to an evaluation by a psychiatrist of my choice. She agreed.

Three months later, she returned with a letter from the psychiatrist in hand. Her surgery was scheduled. Finally, she accepted an appropriately sized implant. In fact, it was the size that was originally suggested to her at her initial consultation. By working with the psychiatrist, she learned that she couldn't accept major changes in her life. To compensate, she chose minor changes instead. Follow-up evaluations revealed her to be quite happy not only with the breast augmentation, but also with her "new life." Most augmentation patients show a marked improvement in their body image that remains stable over time.

A 23-year-old female came into my office to be evaluated for breast pain from cysts in her breasts. She requested removal of both breasts.

The patient had little breast tissue and scattered fibrocystic disease. Her complaints were out of proportion to her physical examination, thereby bordering on a disorder. She'd already had a hysterectomy at this young age after the birth of her daughter, but she was vague on why she'd had her uterus removed.

I asked her to be evaluated by a psychiatrist; she reluctantly complied. I received a phone call from the psychiatrist about six months later. He stated that she was "ready for surgery." I was somewhat surprised that she'd been cleared for surgery. The psychiatrist explained that she had been physically and sexually abused as a young girl and wanted all her "violated" sexual organs either removed (uterus) or replaced (breasts). After having mastectomies and undergoing implant reconstructions, she's still one of my happiest patients.

Can't They See How They Look?

This brings us back to one of Danielle's initial questions at the restaurant in Los Angeles: "Don't people realize that it's bad? Do they not realize how they look?"

What do the people who we'd classify as having had bad plastic surgery see when they look into the mirror? Do they see the unnatural result we see? Do they believe they were a victim of bad plastic surgery? I've discussed this at length with plastic surgeons and psychiatrists. There's just isn't one good answer.

Based on my discussions with several psychiatrists, below are the top three reasons why people don't see what we do:

1. Some psychiatrists feel patients have a distorted view of what looks good. They see celebrities' results and think it's the way good surgery should look. After all, the rich and the famous have enough money to see the best surgeons so their results must be great. We see this in fashion, too. Celebrities embrace the new avant-garde fashion trends and typically have the body to wear them and look good doing it. We all know people who wear every new style. Yet

some people are unaware of just how bad that style looks on their body type, like when someone with large hips wears a pencil skirt or we see large breasts in a crop top. If people are convinced that something looks good, that may account for their desire to look the same way that celebrities look. Unfortunately, bad plastic surgery has become ubiquitous in Hollywood, so if a regular person turns out looking like their favorite celebrity, they are happy with their new look. They believe they look good.

2. Other psychiatrists feel that we never really see ourselves as we really are. We don't have the capacity to view our true image. Instead, the subjective self-image is what's important to each individual. We perceive what we want to or need to see in the mirror. *If we never see our real self, but perceive it to be less than optimal, then any difference we see is judged to be better.* Patients with bad plastic surgery results truly don't see what we see. They see change that they view as better because for them, anything different is better. In the immortal words of Martha Beck, "Although beauty may be in the eye of the beholder, the feeling of being beautiful exists solely in the mind of the beheld."

3. Another group of psychiatrists posit that a "plastic surgery denial syndrome" exists. This idea builds on the weight denial syndrome where people don't realize how much weight they've gained even though they're growing out of their clothes. What patients don't see is the resulting horror wrought by their recent surgery. They don't realize how bad they look to others and will even deny having surgery. Patients have been in my office with a terrible result from a facelift, yet they neglect to document any surgery on their patient questionnaire. One obviously deformed patient was taken aback when I asked why she didn't return to her facelift surgeon. She denied ever having a facelift!

I believe some patients want to look like they've had work done. They don't want to look natural. They want people to look at them. People like this consider any reaction from others to their appearance to be positive. The fact that others notice they had surgery puts them in the same category as their favorite Hollywood celebrity or the wealthy people going into an expensive restaurant. Remember the classmate at the high school reunion.

You'd think plastic surgeons must know when a result isn't optimal or even good. But I've seen plastic surgeons who don't realize they're victims of bad plastic surgery themselves. A plastic surgeon in St. Louis had his eyes done and now they look beady and dishonest. A cosmetic surgeon also in St. Louis had so much filler injected into her face that she looked like a hot air balloon. A nationally recognized plastic surgeon had a facelift that included having fat injected into his face. Afterwards, he was no longer recognized by his own colleagues.

Many plastic surgeons feel, "If you're happy, I'm happy." As long as the patient feels better and has increased confidence, the outward appearance matters less. The psychological benefits to the patient aren't seen by others.

So, the answer to Danielle's question at the restaurant is, "No, Danielle. They don't see what everyone else can see."

Body Dysmorphic Disorder

Body Dysmorphic Disorder (BDD) or "dysmorphophobia" was described in 1891 by Italian physician Enrico Morselli. It's defined as a psychiatric disorder characterized by an excessive preoccupation with a slight or imagined defect in the person's appearance. This causes significant emotional distress and poor psychosocial functioning. It is much more serious than just "seeing things in a 10X mirror." The excessive preoccupation with the perceived "defect" may influence how the person functions in society. Plastic surgery on a BDD patient could make that patient's psychiatric problems worse.

A BDD diagnosis requires the following:

1. There is a preoccupation with an imagined defect in a person's appearance. This is defined as *thinking about the perceived defect for longer than one hour per day.*

2. The preoccupation causes significant distress or impairment in social situations.
3. No other mental disorder accounts for the patient's preoccupation, such as anorexia nervosa or delusion.

BDD occurs in approximately 2 percent of the United States population. It affects more women than men although the difference is narrowing. The incidence of BDD is greater in a plastic surgeon's office and may be as much as 25 percent higher than the general population.

Clinical associations that may accompany BDD include depression, obsessive-compulsive disorder, substance abuse, social inadequacies, and phobias. Some people develop repetitive behaviors to hide the perceived defect, including grooming, picking to correct blemishes, and excessive makeup to cover or correct abnormalities. Significant impairment of the person's social responses also accompanies BDD. This can result in a poor quality of life, which leads to sufferers' functioning below their capacity. Their poor quality of life is similar to someone with a recent myocardial infarction, severe diabetes, or extreme depression.

BDD patients seek isolation in order to relieve their anxiety. They tend to avoid social situations where their "deformities" may be seen and judged. Eighty percent of patients with BDD have suicidal ideations and about 25 percent have attempted suicide. They appear dumbfounded when confronted by their delusions.

It should be obvious that surgery doesn't cure BDD and, in fact, may make matters worse. These patients tend to blame some of their inadequacies on their perceived deformity, and its elimination means the blame must lie elsewhere. Their crutch has been kicked out from under them. They must face their inadequacies as failures within themselves that have nothing to do with their appearance. This increases their isolation and depression and can lead to substance abuse. The BDD postoperative patient is extremely unhappy and depressed.

It's in everyone's best interest to identify the BDD patient prior to surgery. Correcting the alleged defect cannot be done with surgical intervention. A plastic surgeon can assist the patient by referring them to a psychiatric expert. The appropriate therapist can help the patient see their problem more clearly. When the surgeon thoughtfully and kindly acknowledges the patient's underlying problem, often that patient is grateful and even relieved that they are receiving help.

This is one situation where plastic surgeons need to be well educated and sensitive to the disorder. A doctor's first obligation is to do no harm, and this includes protecting patients from themselves.

Chapter 10
Plastic Surgery Providers

- - - - - - - - - - -

A provider supplies a particular service or makes that service available to others. Some providers of plastic surgery are well-qualified, some are less-qualified, and others aren't qualified at all. The less-qualified and unqualified have capitalized on lax laws that allow them to conduct procedures for which they have woefully inadequate (or no) training. While this lack of training might seem to be a sufficient obstacle for these people, the opportunity to provide a service for financial gain may outweigh their concern for their patients' well-being. Unfortunately for patients, having an unscrupulous provider as their "plastic surgeon" can result in life-altering consequences and sometimes even death. The fact that there are enough less-qualified and unqualified people acting as plastic surgeons to create a television show is both frustrating and startling.

Licensed to Kill premiered on the Oxygen Network in 2019 and highlights medical professionals who put their patients into dangerous, high-risk situations. One episode, entitled "Killer Surgeon," exposed an arrogant "cosmetic surgeon" who offered bargain-priced surgeries out of his basement "operating suite." After the death of a patient in his basement, he was charged with second-degree manslaughter, criminally negligent homicide, second-degree assault, reckless endangerment, and falsifying business records. He lost his license and went to prison. Upon his release, he was arrested for the attempted murder of his wife, which landed him back in prison. Despite his numerous felonies, one patient described him as the most charismatic surgeon she'd ever met and felt good achieving her aesthetic goals under his hand.

This chapter details the difference between plastic surgeons who've sustained rigorous, years-long training to become consummate professionals in this field and the growing number of physicians trained in other specialties as well as non-physician providers who act "as if" they're plastic surgeons but lack the education, training, and certifications to fully claim that distinction. Who does your plastic surgery has a profound influence on your result, and knowing this information could even save your life.

Physicians Aren't Interchangeable

Just because someone has "MD" after their name doesn't mean they're qualified to do plastic surgery. Unfortunately, the public tends to believe that all doctors are the same. To match the demand for aesthetic procedures, many doctors not formally trained in cosmetic alterations and enhancements of the human body have made themselves available for these procedures despite not having rigorous training.

A plastic surgeon performs plastic surgery, but unfortunately not all plastic surgery is performed by plastic surgeons.

The news is full of "plastic surgery gone badly" stories. What's rarely exposed in these stories is that the majority of those procedures weren't even performed by plastic surgeons but by less-qualified or nonqualified providers. Patients are the duped masses who see advertisements that seem to claim the competence and the education of a plastic surgeon from these under- and uneducated providers.

Many patients, during their initial consultation with me, are shocked when I explain that their previous consult was with a non-plastic surgeon provider. This leads to them asking many questions, including how they could portray themselves as a board-certified plastic surgeon in their printed material if it wasn't true. Perhaps unsurprisingly, only 13 percent of patients knows there's no law in the United States governing the advertising practices of physicians.[16] Simply put, these providers are playing on the naiveté of consumers.

So just how prevalent are these non-plastic surgeons? According to unpublished data from the New York University (NYU) Langone Health Center presented at the 2016 annual meeting of the American Society of Aesthetic Plastic Surgeons (ASAPS) in San Francisco, California, it's a lot. After doing a Google search for the term "plastic surgeon," they visited these websites to deep-dive into the provider's qualifications. Seventy-five percent of the websites they visited were from physicians who *weren't* board-certified plastic surgeons. That should scare you.

Broken down by specialty, their list revealed:

- 3,075 Ear, Nose, and Throat (ENT) Surgeons (41%)
- 1,275 General Surgeons (17%)
- 1,125 Oral Maxillofacial (OMF) Surgeons (15%)
- 825 Oculo-Plastic Surgeons (11%)
- 750 Dermatologists (10%)
- 225 Family Medicine Physicians (3%)
- 150 Obstetrics and Gynecological Physicians (2%)
- A remainder including Emergency Medicine, Pediatricians, a Urologist, and an Anesthesiologist (1%)

There was even one physician phlebologist (trained in treatment of leg veins) claiming to be a plastic surgeon.

A more detailed look into the above data showed the percentage of physicians *within* certain specialties who were performing plastic surgery outside their scope of practice. Of the non-surgeon providers, all were practicing outside the scope of their board certification.

- 94% of General Surgeons
- 68% of Oculo-Plastic Surgeons
- 67% of Oral Maxillofacial Surgeons
- 50% of Dermatologic Surgeons

- 21% of Ear, Nose, And Throat Surgeons

Only a third of board-certified plastic surgeons came up in their search. Physicians can "practice" plastic surgery because doctors in the United States *aren't required by law to practice only within their specialized fields regardless of board certification.* Doctors may practice medicine *and* surgery if they attain a doctor of medicine (MD) degree, even if they don't complete the additional training needed for board certification. A medical degree, while representing four hard years of medical school, doesn't come close to the training required for plastic surgeons to become proficient in that specialty. Then why would you think any physician graduating from medical school is competent to perform plastic surgery on you? Please ask for plastic surgery board certification and malpractice status of the doctor performing your plastic surgery or injecting your face.

No agency or group in the United States has accepted the responsibility of protecting patients from providers who misrepresent themselves. No consumer advocacy group exists to protect patients. To fill the void, some states are trying to pass laws to require a more explicit definition of "board certification." It's not much better across the pond. In England, The Royal College of Surgeons has urged their government to change present laws to inform the public whether doctors have the right training to do cosmetic procedures, but as of yet, no change has been made.

Your physician's qualifications are so important.

This is what happened to a liposuction patient as reported in a 2011 *Self Magazine* article.[17] The patient's procedure had been marketed as less expensive but more medically advanced. The doctor explained that as the liposuction was being performed, she'd be in an "awake" state, lucid and "in control." She thought she'd be well cared for because the doctor's website claimed a Johns Hopkins education and contained plenty of testimonials and pictures of smiling patients with the doctor.

During the procedure, which was done in the doctor's office, she spent five hours lying on a stretcher while the physician's assistant jabbed at her while he watched a basketball game. The television in the small room was "cranked up loud enough to drown out her cries."

As often happens in these cases, she learned the truth about her procedure and her doctor after her surgery. She learned that this procedure cost a quarter of the regular price of liposuction because he didn't use general anesthesia or an anesthesia provider. He did the procedure in his office, which was an unsafe, unlicensed facility, because the doctor lacked hospital privileges of any kind. His office was stocked with expired medication, including the local anesthesia, and his assistant's medical qualifications were also questionable.

The doctor proved to be a board-certified radiologist (physicians who diagnose and treat disease using X-rays and more advanced radiation equipment). To learn liposuction, he took a two-day training course for which he paid seven thousand dollars. The patient subsequently spent much more to correct the problems caused by this bargain plastic surgery.

There's no question that qualifications matter. Understanding them will assist you in choosing the best, well-trained provider for your procedure *and* help you avoid a tragedy like the story above.

Board Certification: What It Is and Why It's Important

Board certification isn't required to practice medicine in the US. It's elective additional training that provides an even deeper knowledge base for a physician to draw from when working with patients. It also acknowledges the added training the physician had to acquire and their commitment to the ongoing training that's required to claim board certification.

The entity responsible for certifying physicians is the American Board of Medical Specialties (ABMS). "The mission of the ABMS is to serve the public and the medical profession by improving the quality of healthcare through setting professional standards for lifelong certification in partnership with Member Boards."[18] You can learn more about this process at their website, www.abms.org. The ABMS recognizes the following 24 specialty boards as noted below.[19]

Each specialty is preceded by the words "American Board of":

Allergy and Immunology	Orthopedic Surgery
Anesthesiology	Otolaryngology
Colon and Rectal Surgery	Pathology
Dermatology	Pediatrics
Emergency Medicine	Physical Medicine and Rehabilitation
Family Medicine	Plastic Surgery (ABPS)
Internal Medicine	Preventive Medicine
Medical Genetics/Genomics	Psychiatry and Neurology
Neurological Sciences	Radiology
Nuclear Medicine	Surgery
Obstetrics and Gynecology	Thoracic Surgery
Ophthalmology	Urology

The goal of the ABMS is to provide assurance to the public that a physician specialist certified by a Member Board of the ABMS has successfully completed an approved educational program and evaluation process. This process must include components designed to assess the medical knowledge, judgment, professionalism, and clinical and communication skills required to provide quality patient care in that specialty. A board-certified physician has demonstrated skill in a particular field to the satisfaction of medical examiners.

In fulfilling their mission, the ABMS will also coordinate peer reviews of Member Boards' standards and processes. The ABMS sets the professional standard, oversees the application of tests, measures medical qualifications and completeness, and assists the public in assessing the abilities of physician. A member of a medical subspecialty recognized by the ABMS is the "gold standard" to assure the best medical care to a patient.

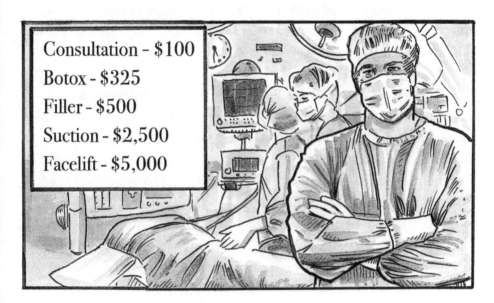

Consultation - $100
Botox - $325
Filler - $500
Suction - $2,500
Facelift - $5,000

The American Board of Plastic Surgery

Being a member of the American Board of Plastic Surgery (ABPS), the only plastic surgery specialty board that's recognized by the ABMS, means a provider can claim the title "board-certified plastic surgeon." The ABPS (www.abplasticsurgery.org), under the watchful eye of the ABMS, sets the standards for physicians to be considered for certification and administers competency testing to ensure understanding and execution of accepted practices within the field of plastic surgery. The ABPS is the only board that certifies the full spectrum of the specialty of plastic surgery of the entire body at all ages and currently recognizes approximately 9,000 board-certified plastic surgeons. *It must be emphasized again that the ABPS is the only plastic surgery board recognized by the ABMS.* As such, facial plastic surgery, cosmetic surgery, and oculo-plastic surgery *aren't* recognized as legitimate boards by the ABMS.

The American Society of Plastic Surgeons

To be a member of the ASPS, a physician must be board-certified in plastic surgery and fulfill continuing medical education presently consisting of a hundred fifty education hours every three years including a minimum number of hours devoted strictly to patient safety. There are about 7,000 members of the ASPS (www.plasticsurgery.org).

The American Society for Aesthetic Plastic Surgeons

The ASAPS is a subspecialty society of about 2,600 board-certified plastic surgeons (www.surgery.org). To be a member, these surgeons must focus 80 percent of their practice on cosmetic/aesthetic procedures, which distinguishes them from other plastic surgeons who perform mainly reconstructive procedures.

I'm a board-certified plastic surgeon (ABPS) recognized by the ABMS. I am a member of both the ASPS and the ASAPS. To achieve my professional education goals, *nine years* of post-medical school training was required. This included six years of general surgery and three years of plastic surgery training. I wanted to give the best care I could to my patients, so I willingly chose this difficult pathway to get the best education possible. This lengthy training, as well as overall experience, makes board-certified plastic surgeons the experts in aesthetic surgery.

Know Your Plastic Surgeon's Background

Plastic surgeons perform plastic surgery but not all plastic surgery is performed by plastic surgeons. It's crucial you keep this truth in mind as you search for your provider. It's to your benefit to understand the training and experience of the person who's going to alter your face or body. And it's imperative you ask questions to get the details on their background! Also keep in mind that if a potential provider seems unwilling or unable to answer your questions, you probably want to go elsewhere.

To determine if a provider is a board-certified plastic surgeon, ask them exactly by whom they are certified or ask specifically in what they are certified. If they say anything other than "plastic surgery," then they aren't a plastic surgeon. In fact, if they indicate "board-certified" without a specialty designation, that may mean the physician is certified in family practice, internal medicine, rehabilitation medicine, or any one of the twenty-four boards recognized by the ABMS—but not plastic surgery. More states need to pass laws requiring providers to state their board certification field and not just say they're "board-certified" or "boarded." This simple piece of information would go a long way in supporting consumer education.

Of course, as the next section will explain, some physicians will claim board-certified status from a board that's not recognized or condoned by the ABMS. This creates even more consumer confusion as they're unable to easily see the difference between legitimate and bogus credentials.

Plastic Surgeon versus Cosmetic Surgeon—What's the Diff?

The power of the term "board-certified plastic surgeon" carries a lot of weight. But for providers who aren't plastic surgeons, the need to appear credentialed was difficult until the creation of the American Board of Cosmetic Surgery (ABCS) in the waning decades of the twentieth century. As you may have guessed, this board isn't recognized by the ABMS nor does it have the strict requirements of the ABPS. What the ABCS does do is provide cosmetic surgeons the *appearance* of the same educational and experiential qualifications of plastic surgeons. A board-certified plastic surgeon already has more experience in cosmetic surgery than any other "boarded" provider who has applied to the ABCS.

What this organization has done is attempt to position all plastic surgeons as reconstruction specialists: that is, we only work on recreating areas of the face and body damaged or destroyed by accident or illness. They position cosmetic surgeons as specialists in all things aesthetic. This simply isn't true. Further, the one-year cosmetic surgery fellowship can't be compared to the required several years-long trainings that board-certified plastic surgeons must take.

What may be even worse (certainly for consumers) is that the fellowship these physicians are enrolled in isn't sanctioned by the Accreditation Council for Graduate Medical Education (ACGME). The ACGME is the governing body in the United States responsible for overseeing and approving graduate medical training programs. The ACGME mandates that after completing an approved residency, that physician is competent in medical knowledge, patient care, and professionalism. Because of its rigorous standards, ACGME accreditation is a driving force behind the high quality of American medicine. Without oversight by the ACGME, the ABCS established their own criteria, qualifications, and acceptable standard of training. As such, there is no existing cosmetic surgery fellowship sponsored by the ABCS that is accredited by the ACGME.

Both the ACGME and the ABMS exist to assure the public that the quality of healthcare in the United States is constantly improving by establishing, assessing, and advancing the professional standards of physicians in their field of medical training. Unfortunately, in a free market society, these professional standards are often challenged by others.

Legal Woes for the ABCS

In 2013, the Utah Board of Plastic Surgery began an ad campaign to increase public awareness that all plastic surgeons aren't created equal. One of their most controversial billboards depicted a crying woman saying, "I Didn't Know My 'Cosmetic Surgeon' Wasn't a Plastic Surgeon." The Board was taken to court by two cosmetic surgeons who alleged anti-competitive practices by the Board. The case was thrown out of federal court.[20] The case was appealed and the dismissal by the court in 2013 was affirmed by the Circuit Court of Appeals in 2015.[21]

In a December 18, 2018, landmark decision, the Medical Board of California (MBC) denied by unanimous vote the ABCS's request to advertise as "board-certified cosmetic surgeons." The MBC reviewed the cosmetic surgery training programs and concluded that the ABCS training programs of a single year couldn't consistently provide the needed broad-based exposure to all aspects of cosmetic surgery. The current

ABCS training programs don't appropriately prepare their trainees and are far less rigorous than what's required for the ABPS certification. This decision should reassert and preserve the public's perception that "board certification" is associated with a physician who delivers the highest quality care to their patients.

A few years ago, I did a search on the ABCS website to see how many physicians in the St. Louis Metro area were listed. At that time, there were eight: three otolaryngologists, two oral surgeons, one dermatologist, one cardiac surgeon, and one oral maxillofacial surgeon. Of those eight, none were board-certified in plastic surgery. A more recent check showed only one provider was listed in the city now, an otolaryngologist.

During my first search, I recognized a name in another city as a fellow who had attended my general surgery training program and gone on to otolaryngology and facial plastic surgery. I asked him why he chose to join the ABCS. He said it allowed him to branch out of his expertise. Now he was able to do breast augmentations and body liposuctions instead of just facial plastic surgery. In other words, he was performing procedures he wasn't initially trained to do in order to bring more patients into his practice. It sounded more like a business proposal and marketing decision than a way to offer the best patient care.

The Board-Certified Plastic Surgeon Difference

The advantages of having a board-certified plastic surgeon care for you are the qualifications and expertise they bring to every patient interaction. Board certification in plastic surgery is training in surgery that takes five to six years to complete. They've been trained and are qualified to care for you from "head to toes and birth to death."

A board-certified plastic surgeon can perform your coworker's hair transplantation and remove a melanoma under the toenail of your best friend. They can repair the cleft lip of your granddaughter and remove the skin cancer on the face of your great-grandfather. That same board-certified plastic surgeon will also be able to perform your facelift as well as care for everyone in your family.

A difference that's frequently mentioned is the cost difference of going to a board-certified plastic surgeon versus other providers. As the identified plastic surgeon at a St. Louis social function, I was approached by a guest who asked me, "Why should I go to a board-certified plastic surgeon when I can go to this new 'cosmetic-trained' physician who recently opened shop and only charges a quarter of what the established plastic surgeon charges me?"

Price is the last thing to consider when searching for a plastic surgery provider. You don't want someone saying the old adage "You get what you pay for" after undergoing a plastic surgery procedure! Please ask questions of your provider to establish board certification, their expertise, and their qualifications. Many cosmetic surgeons depend on the naiveté of potential patients and the perceived "blurred lines" between board-certified plastic surgeons and other providers. If you want a board-certified plastic surgeon to perform your surgery, ask to see their credentials and only accept board certification in Plastic Surgery.

All Other Providers Attempting Plastic Surgery

This category includes other specialty surgeons as well as nonsurgical physicians who perform plastic surgery procedures outside of their board certifications. Make no mistake. These physicians, while likely talented and board-certified in their area of expertise, aren't qualified to do plastic surgery procedures. They depend on patients not knowing the difference between certification by the ABPS and simple board certification in their specialty. They add plastic surgery to their patient offerings usually to increase business and revenue.

The physicians who perform procedures outside the scope of their board certification gain their "knowledge and expertise" through seminars, conferences, or from product manufacturers. The unsuspecting public wrongly assumes that if someone does a procedure, they're qualified to do it. If a physician is trained briefly (e.g., over the weekend) or think they can do a procedure without taking formal training, they may miss the anatomic considerations or surgical nuances that give the best result for the patient. For example, cutting off the skin during closure of a gynecologic procedure looks easy, so it's often attempted by non-plastic surgeons.

A report by the National Surgical Quality Improvement Program found that skin removal or "panniculectomy performed by plastic surgeons results in lower rates of overall postoperative complications compared with that performed by non-plastic surgeons."[22] This means having the procedure done by your gynecologist is more likely to result in complications, which, at the very least, will decrease the aesthetic result of the procedure and may delay recovery. The wife of a plastic surgeon here in St. Louis recently tried to coordinate a tummy tuck with another plastic surgeon and a hysterectomy by a gynecologist. But the gynecologist told her that he could do the tummy tuck for her and do it just as well as the plastic surgeon. That's no different than if I offered a hysterectomy along with a tummy tuck.

Less-qualified physicians do cosmetic procedures because no one tells them they can't do them. In the past, regulators overlooked country doctors who weren't trained to but delivered babies anyway due to the lack of obstetrical care in rural areas. Regulators didn't want to "limit the physician's scope of practice." In a sense, this is how many less-qualified physicians get away with doing cosmetic procedures. But these same physicians are unaware of the possible complications that could arise because their training didn't include oversight by a qualified plastic surgeon who's performed many of these procedures and understands how to avoid and treat complications.

Unless patients delve into a physician's background and credentials, they'll never know the doctor really isn't qualified to perform the procedure. Instead, these uninformed patients will assume the doctor is qualified because they're offering the procedure. Sadly, many patients will go to them because they don't charge the "outrageous" prices that board-certified plastic surgeons charge.

State medical boards do little to regulate procedures and practices in a physician's office. If the procedure isn't performed at the hospital, then there's little oversight. Twenty-five states have no statutes or guidelines for office-based surgery.[23] This means that there are *no guidelines* on what provider can do the surgery, what type of facility the surgery can be performed in, or what type of procedure may be done.

I'm not qualified, but I could, as a Missouri physician, perform any number of procedures in my office, including a heart bypass. The patient, in a situation such as this, is at risk for complications because there are no rigorous training requirements expected of me as the surgeon performing the heart bypass operation. In most states, the provider of office surgery isn't even required to maintain a state license or registration.[24] Only four states (California, Florida, Louisiana, and Texas) require physicians to disclose to their patients their medical backgrounds and board certification. Only a few states even require the provider performing office-based surgery to have staff privileges in a hospital for the performed procedure. More states need to adopt these regulations to protect patients.

Not understanding complications is one thing. Having a lack of concern for the patient's well-being is another. A patient came to see me for some secondary corrective surgery to repair surgery performed in a doctor's office. As instructed by the other physician's staff, she filled a prescription for Valium and then took it on the way to her procedure. Once in operating suite, her face was cleansed with soap and water. Then she sustained over 50 injections of local anesthesia in her face. She felt every one of those needle sticks because the Valium wasn't working well. It finally kicked in for the initial part of the surgery, but halfway through, she was awakened by the surgeon who told her that he and his assistant were "going for lunch." He instructed her not to move because her face was "open." She lay in the chair concerned that at any moment she might expose her "open face" to bacteria or injury. She also desperately needed to visit the restroom.

After a time, the surgeon and his assistant returned from their lunch. Another Valium was slipped into her mouth, and they resumed the procedure. Her husband picked her up around dinnertime. She left with her face in bandages, wondering what in the world had happened to her. She cried as she told me how much pain she was in during the surgery but felt she couldn't complain to the surgeon. It was a humiliating experience for her.

I reassured her that the experience she'd have with our office would be different. More importantly, the corrective surgery would be done in our hospital outpatient operating room under general anesthesia with full monitoring. And no lunch break.

The hospital may, in fact, be the best regulatory board because the hospital reviews cases, complications, and certifications. If you want to be sure a provider is qualified to do your procedure, ask them if they're able to perform that procedure in the operating room in a hospital. Then ask which hospitals they can perform it in.

This question is especially necessary when considering liposuction. Many providers suggest that they can perform liposuction in their office at a lower cost. Their answer to your hospital question will tell a lot about the oversight of their abilities and the response to any complications you might experience. At our hospital, a patient was transferred to our emergency room from the office of a less than qualified provider. The patient had no fewer than ten perforations in her bowel from poorly done liposuction and survived only after multiple heroic lifesaving surgeries by our general surgeon.

Years ago, I was one of three defense witnesses for a local plastic surgeon being sued by a patient for bad scars after breast reduction surgery. The opposing "expert" plastic surgery witness was an Emergency Medicine boarded physician who occasionally did upper eyelid surgery in a friend's office but who had no hospital privileges for any surgical procedure. His "expert" statement as a "plastic surgeon," without any personal experience of breast reduction surgery, was that he "had never seen such bad scars as this lady's scars," which he only reviewed in a photograph. He never once personally saw the patient. Despite his grossly inadequate qualifications, the case was scheduled for trial. The case was dismissed three days before the trial was to start but the plastic surgeon had already incurred thousands of dollars in legal fees.

Less-qualified providers are, unfortunately, a dime a dozen these days. I hope it's clear that you have every right as the patient to ask about your potential surgeon's medical qualifications, hospital privileges, experience with the procedure you're considering, and the training received to do the procedure.

Less-Invasive Procedures and the Less-Qualified Physician

Some of these less-qualified providers, who have no training in surgery much less plastic surgery, are always trying to push the envelope of "less-invasive procedures." They're trying to match the more dramatic results of surgery. Nothing can match the results obtained in surgery—period. But that doesn't mean these providers don't try, often to the detriment of their patients.

A less-qualified provider can only give more of whatever was done initially: more neuromodulator, more filler, hotter lasers, etc. However, more isn't necessarily better. If a patient needs more changes to get a better result, then a board-certified surgeon can offer surgical improvement.

A quick comparison of noninvasive procedures versus their surgical counterpart underscores this distinction.

Noninvasive Technique	Surgical Technique
More neuromodulator leaves the forehead motionless.	A brow lift will raise the eyebrows and eliminate the muscle forces between the eyebrows.
More filler overfills the face.	A facelift and deep fat pocket injections sets the patient back ten years in appearance.
Skin-tightening lasers can be pushed too hard, creating burns.	A mini facelift with light ablative laser resurfacing work together to result in an attractive, youthful face.
More filler in the lower eyelids may become palpable and visible, and it narrows the eyes.	Surgical repositioning of fat and skin tightening eliminates the folds and fills the cheek eye hollow.

Most surgeons see aging as an occasion to lift, reposition, and tighten, whereas most non-surgeons see aging as an opportunity to fill or relax.

We now have "facelift results without surgery" advertised in the media. These include the Dental Facelift, Fractional Laser Facelift, the Ultrasound Mini Facelift, and the Liquid Facelift.

The Dental Facelift promised facelift results with the placement of "facelift dentures." These do nothing more than soften the downward turned corners of the mouth by creating the appearance of the bone that's been lost due to aging and supporting the soft tissues of the mouth.

The Fractional Laser Facelift uses the energy of a fractional laser to stimulate the deep structural support layer of the skin without disturbing the skin surface. The work is all done from inside the mouth. The laser tightens the skin around the mouth, the chin, along the jawline, and under the eyes. It's worth mentioning that the structural support layer is what's typically addressed in a surgical facelift.

The Ultrasound Mini Facelift uses the same energy employed for years to increase the penetration of skin products but now "lifts the skin" by adding more ultrasound energy, which generates heat. The heat produced traumatizes the soft tissue directly below the skin. The body perceives the heat as an injury, causing an inflow of blood and the release of fluid from the cells. Swelling and edema are the result, softening wrinkles and tightening the skin. Add a little filler and the patients look great initially. Post-procedure photographs are usually done at this stage.

But as healing occurs over a few months, the swelling resolves, and the effect of the noninvasive procedure is less dramatic or may even be gone completely. Most people require yearly treatments to maintain any improvement. In the end, a 30 percent improvement with noninvasive procedures employing the ultrasound and RF equipment may be achieved. But the patient might end up spending more money than if they'd undergone a facelift procedure since the noninvasive procedure needs to be repeated to maintain the effect.

Years ago, I attended a conference in Dallas, Texas, to teach plastic surgeons how to do the Liquid Facelift. An injection session was done with a live patient who looked improved; the injections helped tremendously. One conference attendee raised his hand and asked how much filler was placed and what the total cost was for the injectable material. It turned out that the material cost alone was about six thousand dollars. He then asked the obvious question, "How do you expect me to bring her back in one year and charge her another six thousand when a total facelift would cost ten to twelve thousand and last ten to fifteen years?" The room exploded with applause. The presenters responded that this procedure would be for patients who don't want surgery. The attendee who asked the question then retorted, "Well, then she doesn't want a plastic surgeon. She needs someone who can sell her that six-thousand-dollar procedure again in a year!" He sums up perfectly the hidden costs that can occur in noninvasive procedures. Unlike surgery, they don't offer permanent results. Patients must pay repeatedly for a consistent appearance that surgery could create once.

It seems everyone is getting into the face- and body-transformation game. The gynecologist of one of my patients retired, and she was referred to another gynecologist's office. When she signed in at the reception desk, she was handed multiple glossy marketing pamphlets showing that the office did laser body sculpting, ultrasound skin tightening, neuromodulator and filler face injections, hair removal, and laser skin resurfacing. During her wait, she glanced through the brochures. Finally, she walked back to the receptionist and asked, "Does this office even do gynecology exams, PAP smears, and mammograms, or only this stuff?" She held up the pamphlets for emphasis. She elected to leave before seeing the doctor and found another office for her well-woman care.

I think the patient needs to be suspicious when their cardiologist, internist, gynecologist, dentist, or rheumatologist (to name a few) starts offering cosmetic interventions in their office. They say they do it to expand their practices, but it's more likely done to increase revenue to offset declining insurance reimbursements and rising malpractice costs.

Primary care providers have expanded their practice to build profitability by offering such services as neuromodulators, injectables, skin care, lasers, nutrition, and weight loss. Beware when your cardiac surgeon starts offering breast augmentation, claiming he is qualified because he "operates on the chest." We have seen this in St. Louis. Plastic surgeons spend many years perfecting breast augmentation techniques. Once again, it's not as easy as it appears.

Physicians who incorporate noninvasive procedures into their practice need more than a weekend course from the product manufacturer to deliver these procedures and products safely to their patients. These "courses" don't provide adequate training to develop the proper surgical judgment. These "courses" don't teach physicians who's a good candidate for the procedure, what form of anesthesia is the safest, how to avoid complications, and even more importantly, how to react to complications. Since injectable fillers and laser procedures have a high likelihood of potential serious complications, I believe the training in their use should be much longer than the weekend time frame used by Bass Pro Shops to teach bass fishing or a bathroom tile seminar at Home Depot. Don't you agree?

In contrast, board-certified plastic surgeons spend at least five years learning the same things taught to these less-qualified providers in a weekend training course. As part of a mentoring program, I've traveled throughout the country to teach physicians how to inject a new product. I was flabbergasted by the poor injection techniques exhibited by these "skilled" physicians. In fact, I had to stop a number of training sessions because these "experienced" physicians could have caused serious harm to their patients with their poor level of skill and their poor knowledge of the anatomy. A colleague of mine looked at cadaver injections by "qualified and experienced" physicians and found that these injectors missed the appropriate muscle in *over 50 percent* of the injections! Nonphysician injectors missed the appropriate muscle *78 percent* of the time with their injections. Johann Wolfgang von Goethe said it best: "Nothing is more terrible than to see ignorance in action."

I've mentioned this before, but it's worth stressing again. All physician providers take an oath of "Do No Harm" when graduating from medical school—this is called the Hippocratic Oath. When physicians drift into providing cosmetic procedures, usually for the additional revenue, they seem to forget this oath. One such physician told me that the Hippocratic Oath no longer applied because he was providing aesthetic improvement and not real medicine! Some say that it's "just" cosmetic surgery and, therefore, not a big deal.

Ancillary Providers

Another class of less-qualified, or in some cases, unqualified practitioners are ancillary office or spa assistants who often perform many minimally invasive or noninvasive procedures. Some of these ancillary staff include nurse practitioners and registered nurses, but it also includes medical assistants, cosmetologists, and aestheticians. The qualifications of these providers include many different levels of training and knowledge. But with regard to aesthetic procedures, they all receive their education at conferences, seminars, and from the supervising physician. Many ancillary personnel attend a weekend class and then claim they're certified to inject their own patients. A diligent nurse with fifteen years of experience working in an intensive care unit felt ill-equipped to perform injections despite having attended certification classes prior to working in our office.

These ancillary staff may be supervised in a physician's office, but they may also work unsupervised in a medical spa setting performing both noninvasive and minimally invasive treatments. Typically, in physicians' offices, the medical supervisor of ancillary personnel is onsite if issues arise. This isn't the case in medical spas where the overseeing physician is rarely onsite.

Problems arise when the ancillary personnel don't fully understand the proper protocols for the procedure they're doing on a patient. A darker-skinned patient of mine had extremely hyperpigmented squares on her legs after undergoing laser hair removal. The provider didn't understand that darker-skinned people absorb more of the energy than lighter-skinned people, so she used the wrong protocols for this patient. When the patient questioned the provider about her extreme level of pain, she was told that it had to be painful to work. The patient was left with significant scarring on both legs.

Another patient came in with facial scarring after an erbium laser. After questioning the provider, he said he used all the settings the manufacturer had taught him to use, although he admitted the procedure seemed more painful to the patient than he expected. Upon further investigation, it was discovered that the laser output was much higher than the desired energy level dialed in by the provider. Unfortunately for my patient, the provider didn't have the experience to stop the procedure before causing the major burns.

Lawsuits involving laser treatments by ancillary providers are on the rise. Over a three-year period, the percentage of litigation cases involving nonphysician operators increased almost threefold.[25] Ninety-one percent of cases brought against hair removal technology involve these nonphysician providers, and 64 percent of the cases involving nonphysician operators were done in facilities classified as spas or salons. Yes, the procedure is cheaper, but at what cost?

Appropriately, most states consider laser treatments to be the "use of a medical device." State regulations pertaining to the use of a medical device typically requires an initial evaluation by a physician, physician assistant, or a nurse practitioner. In their judgment, the physician or physician substitute may then delegate the laser treatment for that patient to a qualified laser technician.

But who is a qualified laser technician? The person performing the laser treatment should understand laser physics, have received appropriate training on that particular laser, know the effects of that laser, and know exactly what to do if something goes wrong. The technician should also realize that a laser will affect the various skin types differently, and they should know when to stop a treatment based on patient comfort and skin results. Having a "Qualified Laser Technician" certificate on the wall is nothing more than a laser manufacturer attesting to the fact that the person signed into a particular laser training program. Since there's no confirmation of the knowledge obtained through a test or demonstration, the technician may have signed in for credit and then went out for breakfast and a city tour.

A laser certificate doesn't authorize anyone to perform a laser treatment; it just states that the person attended a class or seminar. The same holds true for injectors, too, since neuromodulators and fillers are also considered medical devices.

Always check the credentials of providers in medical spas. When the owners rely on ancillary staff to determine patient acceptability and provide treatment, things can go very wrong, as this next story illustrates.

A St. Louis clinic marketed LipoDissolve, a non-FDA approved fat-dissolving product. In fact, the clinic used the product name as the business name. They promised patients they'd lose fat easily through the product's ability to destroy fat cell membranes and flush the waste out of the body because of the body's inflammatory response. The clinic had two local medical directors, but they were rarely onsite. They depended on physician assistants and nurses for patient evaluations and treatments. These ancillary providers, however, had only received their training during a weekend certification course.

After nearly one and a half years, the center had to close because of numerous lawsuits. The clinic had lax patient acceptance criteria, which meant many weren't good candidates for LipoDissolve. Despite not being good candidates, if they came with a checkbook or credit card, they received the advertised procedure. A number of clients had minor complications and others didn't receive the results they were promised. At least one young female developed gangrene of the abdominal wall, which required multiple surgical debridement procedures and reconstructive surgeries.

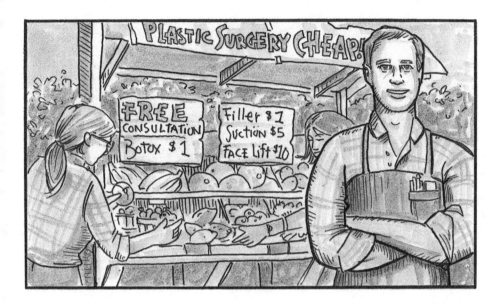

Bargain Providers

In my opinion, the scourge of the less-qualified physicians is those who offer their services at bargain basement prices. They may justify their cost as a means to gain new clients. More often, their pricing correlates to their qualifications and ability to perform the procedures advertised. These are true plastic surgery nightmares. People are dying from back-alley plastic surgery to find a bargain and save money.

The retail mentality shouldn't be applied to aesthetic procedures. Don't have the procedure performed by a nonqualified provider who charges a tenth of what a legitimate provider's services will cost. If you can't afford a legitimate provider, save your money so that one day you can. How can you expect to receive the same quality at a quarter of the price that you would receive from a legitimate physician's practice?

Once the damage is done, it can be tricky to undo. I don't care about what these charlatans charge; I care about the men and women who are duped and harmed by the provider's lack of skill and ethics—all to make a buck. As a patient who came to me for a revision facial surgery consult said, "I was promised the world but sold my face for three thousand dollars."

Sometimes, these bargain providers make headlines for the worst reasons:

- "Lack of training can be deadly in cosmetic surgery" (this article details several cases of misconduct that ended in death for the patients.).[26]
- "Two women dead after liposuction, police say."[27]

Thus far, I've only pointed out physicians who are charging bargain prices for plastic surgery procedures. Sadly, this practice isn't limited to those who hold a medical degree. Completely unqualified, poorly trained laypeople will attempt these procedures. As I've said before, these are dangerous services in the wrong hands. I can't stress this enough: Always be skeptical of cosmetic treatments by individuals not licensed to perform medical procedures.

These headlines bear witness to how horribly awry these procedures can go in the wrong hands:

- "Death of St. Louis County woman highlights risks of illegal buttocks injections."[28]
- "'Dr Lipjob' ordered to stop injecting Botox, impersonating a doctor."[29]
- "The penis and butt surgeries went way wrong. And a fake doctor will pay for it."[30]
- "A Woman got 'lamb fat' injected into her buttocks; now she needs major reconstructive surgery."[31]
- "NJ Woman Pleads Guilty in Man's Death After Penis Enlargement."[32]
- "Man charged with manslaughter in Florida butt-injection case."[33]

These bargain providers put their own greed above their clients' health and safety, and none can justify their training or experience when a patient is injured. Their patients were persuaded by glowing reports by other patients, which often were not true.

An important thing to remember is that unless there's a legal proceeding or a prosecution, rarely do complications end up in the media. When victims of bad plastic surgery survive, their disastrous results are typically not reported due to medical privacy laws in the United States. Unfortunately, this keeps the public ignorant of the dangers of certain providers. Only when a number of patients are injured and complaints are filed to the appropriate authorities are these providers shut down.

Other examples of bargain plastic surgery include plastic surgery clinics at academic institutions, raffles, discount coupons, and being asked to be a "guinea pig" for a new procedure.

Plastic surgery training program clinics would seem like a perfect place to get discounted plastic surgery. After all, these physicians are going to be plastic surgeons one day, so they must be good. This isn't necessarily true. These plastic surgery trainees need to be appropriately supervised by an experienced board-certified plastic surgeon. Some of these trainees are working under supervision, but many are not. While in my academic positions, I've been asked many times by the risk management department of the teaching hospitals to help make an unsatisfied clinic patient happy. These cases were some of the worst ones I've seen, and fixing them truly tested my ingenuity.

Beware of a raffle that promises bargain, or even worse, free plastic surgery. In winning a raffle you have no choice who does your surgery since the surgeon has already been selected. They're usually selected because they want the free advertising. The surgeon also doesn't select you and hasn't been able to evaluate if you're a good candidate for the raffled surgery. You're obliged to have that surgeon operate on you. The surgeon is also obliged to operate on you even if you're a poor candidate for the procedure or are at increased medical risk for complications. These contingencies are usually in the contract and need to be fulfilled by both sides.

Because it's unethical for a member of the ASPS to participate in a "raffle or auction" where there isn't a choice for the surgeon or the winner, the participating surgeons aren't board-certified plastic surgeons most of the time. Winning a breast augmentation in a raffle will almost always mean your surgeon is not a board-certified plastic surgeon.

Discount coupon programs may be ethically problematic in a manner similar to raffles. With online discount programs, the purchaser has no choice as to who will perform the surgery. Also, similar to the problems with raffles, there's no prescreening by the physician to determine whether the purchaser is a good candidate for the procedure.

Being a "guinea pig" is *not* a bargain and only a recipe for plastic surgery disasters. Most people seem very willing to try almost anything for "free," but this is a very risky proposal. Why would anyone want to be a surgeon's first patient for the procedure even if it's done at a bargain price? A surgeon trying their "first" means that they have never performed the procedure before and won't be aware of specific nuances of the anatomy or the procedure. I get a few requests each year to be a "guinea pig" provider for a new procedure. I always decline, saying that I'd never "try" a new procedure on a patient without first perfecting it on cadavers. That way, when I do the procedure on a patient, the patient's no longer a guinea pig but, instead, someone who will receive a properly performed procedure.

Manufacturer Providers

One of the world's biggest lies is "medically proven." This statement usually comes from a company's own research and development department. We've all seen companies promoting the "greatest" product or service and wonder how everything can be the greatest or the best. As a society, we seem to be constantly looking for things that are new and improved, and device manufacturers are more than happy to supply us with the latest and greatest.

But everything can't be the best and greatest. Manufacturers promote their devices directly to the public in the hopes of triggering a patient's request to a provider for that technology. Advertisements for aesthetic services such as the LifeStyle Lift, Botox, Ultherapy, CoolSculpting, etc. appear in magazines, on television, or on online to encourage the public to seek out a provider of those services. Patients need to be aware that the latest and greatest isn't always so.

The marketing and advertising done by device manufacturers is always way ahead of the proven results. To bolster its claims, a manufacturing provider will conduct studies using very few patients and then tout the preliminary results. Make no mistake, these aren't extensive scientific studies. Rarely do the manufacturers take the time to adequately compare the technology and publish the results in a peer-reviewed journal. Publishing in a peer-reviewed journal assures that the research has been put through the rigorous process designed to support the quality and validity of the equipment. It's important to allow the normal scientific evaluation process to continue until large numbers of patients are treated successfully under appropriate study protocols. Studies based on the scientific method would give us a much better idea of the efficacy of the machine or product. But marketing always seems to supersede science in advertising and social media. Unfortunately, because of the lack of science-appropriate testing, a procedure or equipment advertised by the manufacturer as "medically proven" doesn't have the same good connotation as it did many years ago.

Manufacturers also hurry equipment to market by promoting "off-label" uses to other providers. By doing this, they can get the device into the market and in the hands of cosmetic patient providers faster. The manufacturers will also loan the equipment to well-known "consultants" to promote the equipment to others and insist it's necessary to increase patient visits and revenue. Once the devices are in the hands of the providers, the providers must make a ROI to pay for the device and pass the cost down to the patient. Providers seem more concerned about ROI than a patient's results.

Technology Equipment Providers

Lasers are a high-technology item. Manufacturers are quick to market new entrants that often become obsolete in two to three years when the next "latest and greatest" machine is launched.

One such device, at the cost of nearly fifty thousand dollars, was a laser that corrected cellulite deformities. When it first came out, the results were iffy at best, but providers were convinced by slick marketing that they needed one. When it became obvious the results were less spectacular than promised, new anti-cellulite technology replaced the original machine. Although better, it still didn't produce as promised, so still another new machine came out on the market. If a provider purchased each machine, they would have spent about one hundred fifty thousand dollars in total! Despite the newer machines, patients were still unhappy with their results and the providers were unhappy with their ROI. The only people happy in this exchange were the manufacturers who made one hundred fifty thousand dollars from the providers who bought each model. A surgeon I know sold his one hundred-thousand-dollar machine for five thousand dollars just to get rid of it.

Laser liposuction was a marvel of modern marketing directed toward the public. What could be better than combining both laser and liposuction in the same machine? But the marketing and publicity of the machine outpaced the clinical results. A brief hand raising survey of board-certified plastic surgeons at a 2017 plastic surgery meeting in New York City revealed that less than 5 percent of plastic surgeons use laser liposuction. Two thirds of those plastic surgeons who bought the laser say they purchased it for marketing reasons. Potential patients were calling to request the laser liposuction, so they felt obliged to purchase the technology. A number of plastic surgeons claimed, "It was the best dust collector in their office." Two Manhattan plastic surgeons said they kept it in their office for only one week before getting rid of it because it caused heat deformities in the soft tissue. A well-known New York City plastic surgeon claimed that up to 80 percent of his liposuction-revision cases are the result of others using laser liposuction.

Laser liposuction equipment was sold to physicians who believed that the equipment alone predicted the results and that the experience and technique of the operator wasn't important. Because plastic surgeons are no longer interested in the product, it's being promoted for in-office procedures using local anesthesia, which is attracting non-surgeon providers.

Ultrasonic tightening machines, originally marketed to physicians, only one year later were omnipresent in medical spas. I attended a manufacturer-sponsored demonstration of this technology. While the lecturer presented the data, a "volunteer" was presented on the big screen above the presenter. She was undergoing a treatment on her face offstage. At the completion of the procedure, her before procedure photo was placed on the overhead big screen. When she came on stage ten minutes later, the results were outstanding. The audience was then invited onstage for a closer look and to ask questions. But my closer look revealed that the volunteer had several injection sites on her face. A heavy layer of foundation makeup had been used in an attempt to cover them. Her immediate and fabulous improvement was the result of filler injections and makeup done after the ultrasonic treatment and not this "latest and greatest" technology.

Skin tightening using RF was another technology rushed to market by the manufacturers. When it first came out, it was sold to the public as a substitute for a surgical facelift. Physicians, especially non-surgeons, were pressed to get the equipment by public demand. Once all the hoopla settled, both providers and patients were disappointed because the equipment was expensive, the treatments were somewhat painful, and only one third of the patients showed a demonstrable improvement in their appearance or skin tightness. Right on cue, "new and improved" RF equipment was developed and released, promising better results.

A prominent plastic surgeon reported at a national meeting that he spent a quarter of a million dollars on skin-tightening equipment. The equipment was now gathering dust in his closet. He said he only used it on three patients and felt it was a waste of his time and the patient's money. A patient of mine complained that she'd undergone three RF energy treatments at three thousand dollars apiece with another provider with no discernible improvement in her appearance or skin quality. She was surprised when I told her that the equipment was approved by the FDA for wrinkles but not tightening or lifting. Since physicians are using the equipment "off label," the manufacturer is absolved of liability if the results aren't as expected. But physicians aren't absolved of responsibility, and it's in their best interest to represent technology honestly and provide patients with realistic expectations.

As baby boomers age, promoting products that rejuvenate have become common. A case in point is energy-based feminine rejuvenation. Manufacturers have promoted many of the above-mentioned energy technologies (lasers, RF, electromagnetic fields, etc.) to correct gynecological issues such as vaginal laxity, vaginal dryness, pelvic floor muscle laxity, incontinence, and painful sex. These technologies were initially promoted to gynecologists, but the manufacturers found a bigger market by placing the machines in medical spas for a "total body rejuvenation."

The FDA had "cleared" these devices for the treatment of precancerous cervical or vaginal tissue and genital warts. On July 30, 2018, the FDA sent out an FDA Safety Communication to patients and healthcare providers warning that the safety and effectiveness of these energy-based medical devices hadn't been established. The FDA requested that manufacturers stop marketing these devices as claiming the equipment would treat conditions of female genitals, including dryness, pain, laxity, urinary incontinence, and sexual performance. Although these advertisements aren't illegal, the FDA deemed the advertisements as potentially deceptive marketing and felt it necessary to protect the consumer.

Manufacturers also have initiated rewards program similar to airline and credit card company programs. They reward both physicians and patients for using their products. This encourages the patient to ask the physician to use this company's product even though a different product may be more appropriate and work better. It also encourages physicians to use all that company's products because they receive a better ROI by purchasing greater quantities from that company.

Manufacturers stay in business by creating newer and better products. Providers then believe they must purchase these better machines for their patients. Yet the newest equipment often wasn't much better than the old. An honest laser engineer confessed to me that many five- or ten-year-old lasers give the same results as any new and improved version. The older laser may deliver less energy, thus requiring more treatments or a greater number of laser passes, but it would eventually achieve the same result.

Breast Implant Manufacturers

One of the biggest disappointments for me as a plastic surgeon has been the continuing disregard for patient safety by breast implant manufacturers. Prior to 1992, silicone and saline breast implants were popular, although silicone had the edge due to its natural look and feel. Yet silicone implants posed a problem because they ruptured easily. After many lawsuits arose, the FDA, in 1992, advised that silicone implants should only be used for reconstruction after surgery or to correct congenital defects. General use was discouraged. This opened the door for saline implants to take over the market. It also allowed a new entrant, at least in Europe—soybean oil-filled implants.

Marketed under the name Trilucent, these implants appeared to be the perfect answer for breast augmentation. In addition to a more natural look and feel than saline implants, the oil-filled implants magnified breast abnormalities during mammography. In contrast, silicone gel implants obscure about 10 percent of the breast tissue on mammograms.

While women in Europe could get these implants, the FDA in the US kept them under a limited trial to determine their safety and reliability. It didn't take long for issues to emerge. In the human body at a Fahrenheit temperature of 98.6 degrees, the oil became rancid and women were getting sick, especially when the implants ruptured. Implant removal was recommended throughout Europe, and the FDA ordered all implants in the US to be removed to prevent future illness and potential death.

In 2010, a French breast implant company, Poly Implant Prostheses (PIP), was found to be distributing faulty implant devices. Silicone implant manufacturers are supposed to use medical-grade silicone because the impurities inherent in silicone have been processed out. But the PIP silicone implants were discovered to have been filled with a mixture of agricultural- and industrial-grade silicone, which were cheaper than using medical-grade silicone. These implants were found to be more likely to rupture, and many patients became quite ill. It was reported that as many as three hundred thousand women in sixty-five countries had the PIP implants. Since the FDA allowed only a limited trial of these implants, women in the US weren't affected. I have, however, personally removed PIP devices implanted in US patients. The PIP implants were pulled from the market, and the president of the company was fined and sentenced to prison.

Textured implants designed to adhere to surrounding tissues to prevent implant repositioning come with an ominous side effect: breast implant-associated anaplastic large cell lymphoma (BIA-ALCL). At least four hundred fifty-seven women have developed the disease, and nine have died since this type of non-Hodgkin's lymphoma, a cancer of the immune system, was reported in 2011.

In my view, Allergan, the manufacturer of this implant, were slow to stop production and distribution of these implants after their link with cancer was discovered. In July 2019, the FDA strongly encouraged the company to voluntarily recall and remove all non-implanted implants, but this was months after the FDA disclosed an increasing number of lymphoma cases associated with the implant. In May 2020, the FDA warned that the recalled breast implant safety studies were inadequate, and in June 2020, Allergan began to contact implant patients who may not have been aware of the July 2019 recall. Before this campaign by the company to notify patients—almost a year after the FDA recommendations to remove the implants—contacting patients had been left up to plastic surgeons.[34]

Personally, I prefer using products manufactured in the United States, and the only US implant manufacturer is located in Dallas, Texas. I like the idea that the FDA can walk into their manufacturing facility at any time to inspect the quality of the implants that will go into my patients' bodies. This inspection isn't possible with the two other breast implant suppliers, whose implants are manufactured in Costa Rica and Brazil.

FDA-Approved versus FDA-Cleared

The FDA only "approves" drugs and highly technical lifesaving or life sustaining devices. Therefore, "FDA approved" means that the federal agency has concluded that the benefits outweigh the potential risks of a product's intended use. It doesn't mean that rigorous testing has been done to confirm efficacy. It also doesn't mean that safety or effectiveness of the medical device is guaranteed.

Cosmetic devices and injectable material into the skin aren't considered lifesaving or life-sustaining devices. These "Class 2" devices can only receive the designation of "FDA cleared" to be used on humans. What FDA cleared means is that these devices are "substantially equivalent to similar products already on the market." It doesn't mean they are better than what is already being used. Many manufacturers recognize that most consumers don't know the difference between these designations and will market their Class 2 devices such as skin lasers as "FDA approved." This is, without question, wrong.

In fact, the FDA doesn't do its own testing but reviews the studies and tests submitted by the manufacturers. In this way, the FDA determines whether the device is similar to something people are already using but doesn't indicate whether those products or devices actually work better. It's important to understand that an "innovative device" with "FDA approval" may not be any better than other devices on the market. It may not even match the results seen with less-invasive and less-expensive technologies.

Unscrupulous producers have even brought "knockoff" devices into the cosmetic market. These counterfeit machines violate international patents, bypass FDA clearance, and may be appealing to providers because of the lower initial cost, which will give them a greater ROI. Although rare in board-certified physician offices, these knockoff machines are frequently appearing in less-qualified physicians' offices and medical spas. Unfortunately, the risks of injury or an adverse event are much higher with these devices than when a legitimate device is employed. The oversight during production of these devices is poor, and many don't have the same safety features required in FDA-reviewed devices.

Up to this point, the discussion has been on providers in the US. But more and more people are traveling to far-flung locales to have aesthetic procedures done, usually at a much lower cost than in this country. But there are many caveats to medical tourism.

Chapter 11
Medical Tourism

- - - - - - -

G loria only wanted her "mommy makeover" surgery to be cheap. She also wanted to tell her friends that she was going to Mexico for a vacation. The details as to who did the surgery, what the procedure was, and where it was done weren't important to her. She was referred to her doctor by friends in Mexico who assured her that he was wonderful. She saw her doctor the morning of surgery in the operating room inside his office suite. She returned to the US in critical condition with multiple infected areas on her body and a breast implant that kept falling out of the incision in her chest.

Medical tourism is increasing among US residents in almost the same numbers as general cosmetic surgery numbers here. In fact, medical tourism is estimated to be a multibillion-dollar-a-year business. As the name implies, medical tourism means taking a trip to a foreign country to have some type of cosmetic surgical procedure performed.

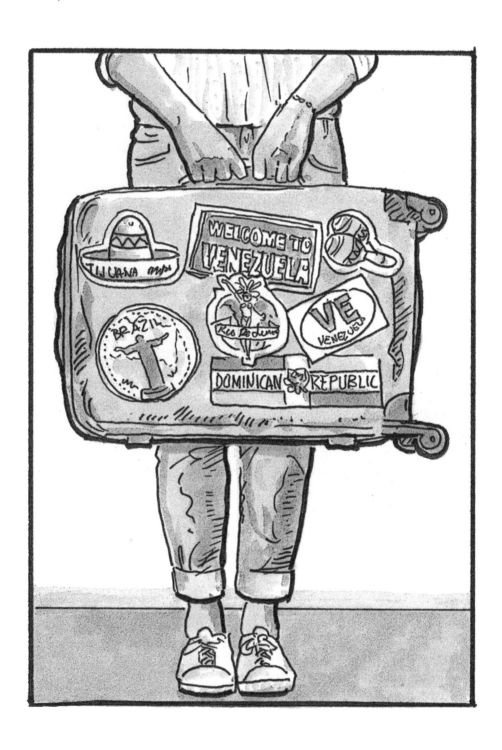

Medical tourism isn't new. Since the 1960s, it's been common for patients wanting anonymity to have their cosmetic procedures performed in Italy, France, England, or Brazil. In fact, a well-respected destination for cosmetic surgery was an island off the mainland of Brazil where a patient could fly in a few days before their surgery to relax and enjoy their surroundings. After surgery, the patient would spend time recovering in a beach house, watching the sunrise over the Atlantic Ocean, drinking champagne, and being cared for by a nurse. As you might imagine, this "destination surgery" is expensive.

Today, medical tourists can now take advantage of cheaper surgery and hospitalization costs (as much as 50 percent less than in the US) in less developed countries. Patients from the US overwhelmingly seek care in Mexico or the Caribbean, but Thailand and the Middle East are also becoming popular destinations. Patients pay in other ways for the lower costs, however.

Instead of a swanky island resort, patients are lodged in a cheap hotel room. Their surgery is performed in a medical facility, often with insufficient emergency equipment or staff. Recovery is done in their sad hotel room with minimal care provided to patients who've just undergone major surgery. A single, postoperative visit occurs about two days after surgery. After that time, patients are on their own. This is unfortunate since complications typically set in at about one week after surgery when the patients have already returned home. Many times, these complications can be severe, even life-threatening. With their surgeon no longer available, patients must find someone to help them, like the patient who visited South Korea for liposuction and presented with dead skin and abdominal muscle in her gynecologist's office. Her doctor was wise enough to refer this patient to my office.

Another patient referred to me had over two liters of bloody fluid in her abdomen and a large necrotic area of dead abdominal wall. She'd been home ten days after undergoing a cosmetic medical procedure in the Caribbean. It was a real deal—she paid five thousand dollars for a procedure that would typically cost about sixteen thousand in the United

States. Well, it would have been a great deal except for all the post-surgery complications care she needed that her *insurance company likely wouldn't cover*. Almost every board-certified plastic surgeon I know has treated patients with complications from procedures performed in medical tourism destinations.

Understand that medical tourism is a foreign industry with much lower surgical standards than the US and little or no oversight. Physician offices and surgical suites in these countries may compromise or even ignore recognized quality and safety standards that exist in the United States. There may be no organization responsible for monitoring these facilities. There are likely no privacy laws in other countries unlike the US, which has the Health Insurance Portability and Accountability Act (HIPAA). This means identities and pertinent information may not be protected.

This leads to the ethical issues of medical tourism. Informed consent is a real concern as patients often meet the staff the day before surgery for their preoperative evaluation and the surgeon only on the morning before surgery. Continuity of care is the physician's responsibility, and foreign physicians often release the care of their patients to others. No communication between the foreign physician and a US-based physician occurs as is required in the US. In many of the medical tourism countries, there's little government regulation or oversight. Medical tourism companies aren't regulated at all.

In 2009, the wife of a rhythm and blues singer suffered cardiac arrest as she was being anesthetized prior to a liposuction procedure in Sao Paulo, Brazil. She was revived but put into a medically induced coma and placed in the intensive care unit for a day. She was transferred the next day to a larger, better equipped facility to recover. She was released from the hospital eleven days later.[35] In the US, most plastic surgeons wouldn't have considered her a candidate for this surgery since she'd given birth to her second child only two months before. They would have insisted she return to her prepregnancy weight prior to any procedure and wait until at least six months after delivery. This obviously was less of an issue for the Brazilian physician and may be why she went to Brazil for the procedure.

The Dominican Republic promotes itself as the choice for medical tourism due to lower costs and medical facilities on par with the US. It's believed that over half of the cosmetic surgeries performed in the Dominican Republic are on patients from other countries. But are the cost savings worth the increased risk of potential complications and poor postoperative care? *In one month*, three Americans died in the Dominican Republic while undergoing or immediately after plastic surgery procedures.[36] As in the US, many providers in the Dominican Republic who aren't certified by the country's Plastic Surgery Society perform cosmetic surgery. They practice in obscurity and operate without regulations or oversight.

In 2016, the Centers for Disease Control (CDC) released a warning to all US practitioners that a large number of patients were returning to the United States with severe infections after having surgery abroad. Some patients had open wounds, abscesses, and skin loss. Ten patients contracted mycobacterium skin infections, the same organism that causes leprosy and tuberculosis, and developed abscesses after cosmetic surgery procedures done at the same surgery center in the Dominican Republic.[37] These infections required hospitalization, removal of dead tissue, and several weeks of intravenous antibiotics upon their return to the United States. The estimated cost to treat these complications was *almost twenty thousand dollars* which more than balances the cost savings of the medical tourism trip.

A nearly five-year study was conducted by researchers in the United Kingdom to better understand the true medical cost of complications from patients who seek cosmetic surgery outside of the UK. The researchers calculated the total cost to the hospital (National Health Service) was almost half a million dollars with an average cost of sixteen thousand dollars per patient.[38]

Uncontrolled bacterial infections raise concern regarding the sterilization techniques used and the quality of the sterile products (instruments, irrigations, and dressings) used during surgery. A plastic surgeon colleague treated a patient who underwent a thread facelift in Thailand who required treatment for a severe infection in the face. The offending bacteria were mycobacterium, the same bacteria discovered in patients having surgery in the Dominican Republic.

Many foreign facilities are actively trying to attract medical tourism by reassuring potential patients that they're accredited by international organizations with a formal agreement between the foreign medical facility and American medical institutions and universities. They also openly recruit Western trained and certified physicians who use the opportunity to be a "medical provider tourist" to a vacation destination. By working this way, patients have doctors who are highly trained and operating in institutions sanctioned by US institutions. But will these US physicians be liable for any complications resulting from the surgeries they perform in a foreign country? Will their malpractice provider cover them for procedures and complications occurring in substandard facilities?

These are all considerations which you must take into account when you're considering going to a foreign country to have cosmetic surgery. Here are some questions I'd like you to think about before you book your surgery and your flight.

- Would you hire an attorney to represent you if they hadn't passed the bar exam?
- Would you hire a plumber to fix your electrical problems?
- Would you hire a construction company to build your house if they weren't bonded and insured?

I'm hoping you answered "No" to the above questions.

The way I see it, medical tourism makes a lot of money for the doctor and the facility in a foreign country. What it often does as well is leave patients sick with complications that could have been easily avoided if the surgery had been done in a US hospital by a competent, board-certified plastic surgeon.

Chapter 12
Pictures, Testimonials, and the Web

- - - - - - - - - - - -

Both qualified and nonqualified providers frequently use pictures and testimonials to dupe the public. Before the internet, plastic surgeons were sent referrals because of the plastic surgeon's experience and credentials. Every patient was a walking testimonial and advertisement for a surgeon's practice. Back then, plastic surgeons couldn't choose only the best results to show to others and hide the ones that weren't so great. Every postoperative patient was a walking testimonial.

Photograph Manipulation

Providers can now choose the photographs they want to show on their website, but more often than you might think, these photos are altered in some way to highlight perceived results. In addition, companies exist that sell flattering (and often misleading) photographs of "patients" that doctors can buy for their websites. I had one of my post-nasal surgery patients appear as a local competitor's result. She was a model and her pictures were selected and purchased for an advertisement layout by that surgeon. Photographs can also be stolen from other sites to display as a provider's result. The internet has given us many wonderful tools, but it's also made it much easier for unscrupulous providers to fool the public.

The most important photographs in the plastic surgery industry are the pre- and postoperative photographs so prevalent on practitioners' websites. I will caveat that many providers show photographs that are true before-and-after images. But others buy photos or alter the photos to emphasize certain features.

Amateur Photoshop manipulations are usually easy to recognize because the jewelry, hair, and clothing are the same for the before-and-after photos, and yet the post-procedure results shown are incredible. Outer contours, so critical for illustrating liposuction results, are easy to manipulate with a dark black background, especially for before-and-after liposuction examples. If you're unsure if what you're looking at is altered or not, zoom in and look at the contour edges. If you see pixilation or fuzziness, it's quite likely that the photo has been manipulated.

Besides manipulations with Photoshop, there are other technical ways to improve results. Results can be faked by managing the light and shadows and the physical pose of the patient. This technique is used extensively in exercise and weight loss advertisements. Technical maneuvers to make postoperative photographs look better include tilting the head back or forward to change the length of the nose or the amount of skin in the neck. Raising the arms will improve the results seen after tummy tucks or liposuction because this maneuver pulls and tightens the torso skin. To make someone look aged, only ambient overhead lighting is used for the "before" shot and a light flash is used for shooting the post-procedure photograph to remove surface irregularities like wrinkles and eliminate shadows. A single-sided flash will cause shadows, but a double-sided flash eliminates the shadows and smooths the skin.

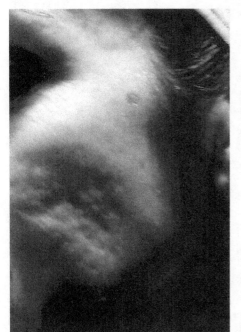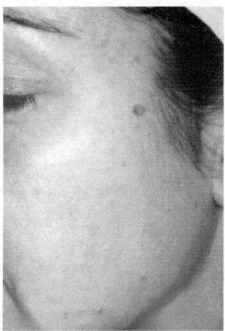

Where the light comes from in a photograph makes a huge difference. As an extreme example, the patient on the left has a deep contour deformity of her left cheek requiring filler for correction (lighting from behind and above patient). Photograph on the right is taken one second later with a camera mounted flash and shows complete correction of the defect with the "latest and greatest filler."

Crow's feet on the outside of the eyes miraculously disappear and appear with animation.

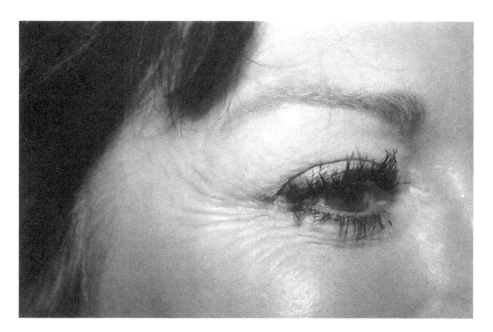

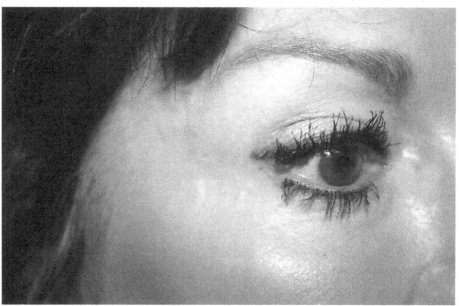

"Before-and-after" photographs reveal a "great result" with skin care products alone. Actually the photographs were taken one second apart with the model no longer smiling and animating. The manipulation is frequently used if the photograph only shows the patient's eyes and not the mouth.

Be especially critical of preoperative photographs without makeup and postoperative photos with makeup. Postoperative makeup may be misleading and used to highlight the good changes after surgery. As we learned from Danielle, the Hollywood makeup artist and hairdresser, well-applied makeup can correct deformities up to five millimeters, which is well over the one millimeter that the human eye can discern. Photographic manipulation and good makeup application can influence postoperative "results" and mislead consumers.

Manufacturers are also sources of photographs.

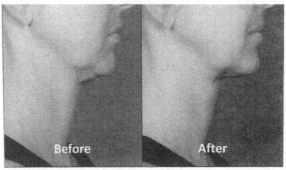

Figure 4. A before-and-after image from the Kybella FDA trials, lateral view.

state that compression makes them more comfortable the first night. All patients will experience swelling, which progresses overnight to an edematous "wattle." This lasts about 48 hours. Most patients will have some bruising and describe their discomfort as mild to moderate. There may

approval, Kybella patients reported moderate improvements after 12 weeks, but as we gain experience with dosage, we will likely see more substantial results. ■

Ed note: This is a brand-new treatment. The author does not have personal before-

Goodbye Double Chin

If you suffer from a double chin, you're not alone!
The American Society of Dermatologic Surgery says 68% of consumers are bothered by their double chin, which can make them look older and heavier.

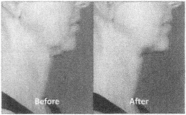

now offers kybella™, the first and only FDA-approved injectable drug that contours and improves the appearance of moderate to severe submental fullness, sometimes referred to as "double chin."

Your double chin may be caused by aging and genetics, and no matter how much you diet or exercise, it may not go away. An injection of Kybella™ can destroy those fat cells and give you a contoured and improved appearance.

Manufacturers sell patient photographs for provider use. The provider in (A) acknowledges the photos in his ads are not his patients. The provider in (B) makes no attempt to inform the public that the photos in his ads are not his patients but lets the public assume that the photo shows his outcomes.

Laser companies, filler manufacturers, and other aesthetic vendors distribute photos to help providers convince patients to use the newest and greatest equipment. These photos are also used to convince a provider to buy the latest and greatest equipment. Many providers and patients can't discern real, unretouched photos from those that are manipulated. The vendors target unsuspecting providers by showing unrealistic results and, in turn, the providers show these unrealistic results to potential patients. The provider wants a good ROI; the patient wants the fabulous result. Often both are disappointed.

Testimonials

The web has made obtaining testimonials easier than ever. But in the world of cosmetic surgery, take those testimonials with a grain of salt because sometimes those testimonials and ratings are coerced or even made up. Case in point: A plastic surgery marketing group has recommended that plastic surgeons place a computer in the waiting room and the office staff should recommend that postoperative patients leave a testimonial and review the physician on a number of ratings websites *before* their postoperative visit.

In 2009, then New York Attorney General Andrew Cuomo fined the LifeStyle Lift company for marketing that was "cynical, manipulative, illegal and knowingly deceiving patients".[39] The company had allegedly engaged in "astroturfing," by having employees fabricate online testimonials as though they were real patients.

The term astroturfing is used when special interests disguise their identities to post online testimonials with the intent of fooling the reader into believing an independent person is writing the comment. Astroturfing gives the impression that there's widespread support for a product, procedure, or piece of equipment through positive comments and testimonials meant to sway consumers' buying behavior. Reverse astroturfing occurs when businesses and providers write unfavorable posts to affect a competitor's business, as when another surgeon or their staff place negative reviews to negatively impact another surgeon.

According to the press release from the attorney general's office, internal emails "show that LifeStyle Lift employees were given specific instructions to engage in this illegal activity. One email to employees said: 'Friday is going to be a slow day—I need you to devote the day to doing more postings on the web as a satisfied client.' Another internal email directed a LifeStyle Lift employee to 'Put your wig and skirt on and tell them about the great experience you had.'"[40]

The Lifestyle Lift company was fined three hundred thousand dollars by New York State. In 2015, the company closed all their offices, declared bankruptcy, and left many patients seeking care for complications from the procedure.

The headline for an antiaging cream advertisement disguised as a "report" made a bold claim that the cream worked so well, a woman over seventy could use it and avoid a facelift. Before and-after-photos showed an impressive improvement in her skin appearance and tightness. Two patients came into my office for surgery and complained that they saw no improvements after using this product for several months. After a quick scan of the forty-four positive testimonials on the product website, I had a hunch that astroturfing was in play. As a counter to all the positive postings, and to prove my hunch, I submitted a diplomatic comment as a physician mentioning that my two patients saw "variable" results. My comment was never included on their website.

Another skin care product employed a different tactic to attract buyers. It used a headline sure to get women's attention as it mentioned an abandoned woman and a fast trick to avoid Botox. Even more intriguing was the first line of the ad, which appeared to be written by a real person who actually lived in St. Louis. The ad went on to promote an antiaging skin care treatment. At the end was a surprise disclaimer in tiny print. It basically stated that the person mentioned in the ad wasn't real and that the results were illustrative of what a user might achieve but weren't guaranteed. The advertiser was counting on women not reading the fine print, and their hopes were well founded. A number of patients mentioned the product to me, didn't read it completely, and spent a lot of money on a product that didn't deliver.

The World Wide Web

Billions of dollars are spent yearly on social media advertisements to sway the public's thinking through subliminal messaging, which tends to influence their choices. Some of these messages include "bargain prices," "procedures with no downtime," and "immediate results." Providers are described using vague adjectives that include experienced, qualified, committed, innovative, and "tops in the field."

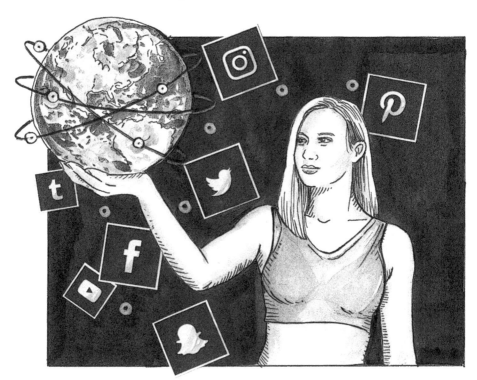

Healthcare marketing is big business. Plastic surgeons are told to "ignite your social media presence and enhance your online footprint." We're encouraged to establish, manage, and protect our online reputations through our social media presence. I had contact with a marketing service whose representative told me up front that she had no experience in healthcare marketing. She said that made no difference because all marketing is consumer and not provider driven. Consumers are looking for attention-grabbing, pleasing colors and ad layouts that "educate" in a few brief lines. Some marketers convince plastic surgeons to promote themselves in highly visible but less than ideal places. This includes shopping mall kiosks, roadside billboards, and even shopping bags and shopping carts.

One of the lectures I attended at a plastic surgery conference stressed marketing and how to run and effectively market your office. The bottom line was: *In today's competitive climate, it is not about the surgery as much as it is about marketing and the business of surgery.*

I couldn't disagree more.

This type of advertising means spending money and time. But what's actually accomplished with all this time and money? A Gallup poll reported that just 5 percent of US residents said social media had a "great deal of influence" on their nonmedical purchasing decisions.[41] A majority of those polled said social media had no influence at all.

Social media is a digital tool that allows its user to share information and content with the public via virtual communities and networks. This means you can put something out on a social media platform, and in theory, billions of people can find and see it. Social media platforms encompass: Facebook, YouTube, WhatsApp, Messenger, WeChat, Instagram, Tumbler, TikTok, X (formerly Twitter), Snapchat, and Pinterest, as well as others. Most marketers feel social media provides a better ROI than other marketing including print and billboards.

The use of social media in plastic surgery is used more frequently than in nonmedical decision making. Over 50 percent of patients seeking plastic surgery used some form of social media, and the most common resource was Instagram (58 percent).[42] The millennial generation used social media the most (77 percent) and baby boomers used it the least (zero percent). All other generations (Generation X and Z) accounted for approximately 20 percent. But only 18 percent of the surveyed patients used a plastic surgeon's social media and/or internet site to resource their proposed procedure.

Chapter 13
The Evolution of Plastic Surgery

- - - - - - - - - - - -

O ver the 30 years I've performed plastic surgery, there have been more changes in procedures than at any other time. In the late 1980s, there were a dozen main textbooks on aesthetic plastic surgery and one leading monthly journal, *Plastic and Reconstructive Surgery*, and a second new monthly journal, *Annals of Plastic Surgery*. We kept up to date in late 1980s and early 1990s by attending conferences and asking the presenters questions. During those years, the conferences were smaller and more intimate. You could actually grab a cup of coffee with a presenter to go into more detail about what was presented.

But a "shared cup of coffee and ideas" is no longer the norm. Memberships in the plastic surgery societies are now much larger. The meeting committees now encourage plastic surgeons to "visit the exhibits" and "promote the corporate sponsors" during lunch and coffee breaks. Medical conferences are starting to resemble trade shows.

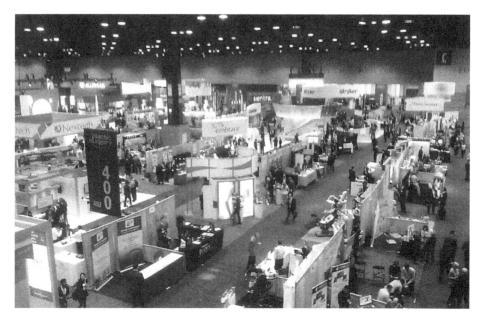

The exhibit hall at a recent meeting of plastic surgeons is where companies may promote the "next greatest thing" to the members.

Manufacturers now have the opportunity to promote their wares: the "newest and the greatest." It's at these conferences that plastic surgeons fulfill their own FOMO by reviewing all the latest lasers, equipment, technologies, garments, skin cream, and office supplies. After a presentation, plastic surgeons can peruse the booths in the exhibit hall filled with providers trying to carve out their place in the booming potential cosmetic patient market.

During the scientific sessions, new procedures are presented to the audience. In the "old" days, long-term patient follow-up after a procedure was at least ten years. Today, two years is considered adequate, but not really enough time to fully evaluate a procedure's lasting results. I personally know many plastic surgeons who, after evaluating their own ten-year follow-ups, no longer perform the procedure that they presented and highly promoted years ago. They found that these new procedures couldn't stand the test of time or were no better than other techniques. I have to remind many younger surgeons that the half dozen cases the presenter shows are their best results. They don't show mediocre or bad results, and they often show the same results repeatedly.

Unfortunately, some surgeons, after viewing these presentations, hurry home to try them out on their significant others and their patients. I've seen some of the worst complications on plastic surgeons' partners. Instead of practicing these new operations in a more forgiving environment, such as anatomy lab or with surgical simulators, they jumped right in and began performing them on their partners and patients. These procedures can't be learned from a ten-minute presentation at a national meeting.

Once, I was called down to the operating room by the nursing staff to help a surgeon who couldn't remember how deep his dissection was supposed to be during a deep plane facelift that he saw presented at a recent meeting. Unfortunately, he was working in the "forbidden" zone where the main nerves are located and where high potential complications could occur. I steered him away from that area, and I stayed to assist with the other side of the facelift. The patient had an early nerve weakness on the initial side but it resolved completely within a month. The final facelift result was one of good symmetry.

Fitting the Patient to the Procedure

Sometimes plastic surgeons are so eager to try a new procedure that they "fit the patient to the procedure" instead of letting the patient's complaints and deformities determine the procedure. While the new technique may not be good or bad, it should be used on the right patient. A well-known plastic surgeon had developed a unique facelift procedure that he presented at all the major conferences. Surgeons were coming from around the world to watch and learn from him. At first blush, the procedure seemed appropriate for everyone. Confidentially, he told me he was performing this procedure on only about 10 percent of his patients. The other 90 percent weren't good candidates. I'm certain that many of the surgeons at his education sessions started doing the procedure on poor candidates, thinking it would work for everyone. As a precaution, always ask your surgeon why they think the procedure they've selected is the best for you, especially if it is unique or innovative.

Sometimes Older Is Better

I paused to listen to an unidentified, older plastic surgeon who approached the microphone after a panel describing new facial procedures at a national meeting in San Francisco. His frustration was evident:

> I have been performing facial rejuvenation surgery for almost 30 years. My facelifts are done by a tried-and-true method giving excellent results. If I changed my way of performing a facelift based on every new idea presented at these meetings, I would be risking my good results and reputation for the sake of joining the latest and greatest. Just because you think it is new doesn't make it better in any way. Your procedures are in total contrast to the procedures that have resulted in very happy patients in my practice over the last 30 years.

Many excellent surgeons get superb results employing classic procedures and forgoing the latest and the greatest techniques. And some classic procedures have enjoyed a reemergence. Many years ago, I was present when a well-known and respected Southern California plastic surgeon made a presentation to a national audience. He presented his results resurrecting a procedure that included an extensive movement of fat under the skin and the resection of skin. The audience almost mocked him and his procedure as old-fashioned and passé. He did his presentation when most national presenters were recommending small skin incisions, slight skin removal, and minimal work under the skin. Seems he was ahead of his time. At a more recent national conference highlighting different perspectives, over 60 percent of the presenters were doing extensive movement and repositioning of fat under the skin and wide skin removal. This just goes to show that when a pendulum swings in one direction, it will swing back.

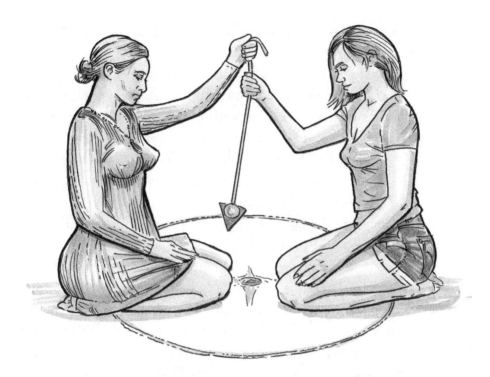

They say plastic surgery is an "evolution of techniques." I think plastic surgeons are sometimes moving "forward to the past." Today's plastic surgeons have returned to firmer and more cohesive silicone breast implants similar to those that were used in the 1960s. Liposuction techniques are now a more mechanical removal similar to the late 1980s and less heat based as was used in the 1990s to melt the fat prior to extraction. Many plastic surgeons are returning to the use of cheaper chemical peels, choosing to leave their expensive lasers in the closet.

A board-certified plastic surgeon has devoted the time to learn the classic procedures during their structured and supervised five years of training, often from surgeons with decades of experience. They'll learn the indications and the anticipated results from the most widely used procedures and how to evaluate each patient as a potential candidate for each procedure. With this solid background in the classics, they'll understand how each surgical procedure began, understand how each has evolved over time, and anticipate the expected results. The breast reduction surgery

I perform today is a combination of techniques used by three different plastic surgeons.

However, there's always room to make procedures better, which is where the nuances of plastic surgery come in. It's also why it's important for every plastic surgeon to keep up with innovative techniques. Sometimes, changing small things will improve the overall technique, producing a better result for the patient. Innovations shift the swing of the pendulum. As innovators, plastic surgeons are always seeking the greatest procedure for each individual patient.

Although pushing the innovation envelope can lead to useful breakthroughs, it can also lead to bad plastic surgery. Sometimes the analysis of the problem is flawed, creating an unnatural and too-done look after aesthetic surgery. An example is how to best reverse the aging process. During aging, plastic surgeons have long believed that gravity acts in a downward force, meaning everything needs to be "lifted." This concept has influenced brow lift, eye lift, cheek lift, facelift, breast lift, arm lift and thigh lift surgeries. In reality, most structures don't need so much to be lifted but, instead, repositioned. Lifting on the vertical can actually contribute to an unnatural result. With a straight upward "lift" there can be a loss of the natural harmony in areas such as the face, trunk, or extremity.

Often, the basis of the procedure is correct, except the nuances that would make it better are missed. The pull on the skin during a facelift probably shouldn't be straight up but should resemble the loss of gravity when the patient is lying flat face up. The skin resection in a tummy tuck should be downward, and the skin removal in a thigh "lift" should actually decrease the circumference of the thigh and *not* lift the skin. It's all about nuance.

A recurrent theme in bad plastic surgery is "a little is good, so more is better." However, keeping the result natural means thinking that "sometimes a little is good and a lot is not."

Not Listening to the Patient

In medical school, physicians learn that the patient will tell the doctor the diagnosis if the doctor truly listens to the patient's complaints and symptoms. If the doctor listens, the patients will tell them what they want from surgery.

Problems occur when a surgeon doesn't listen to the patient and doesn't understand their needs. They try to fit a patient to the procedure and not the procedure to the patient. At a national meeting, a plastic surgeon pontificated by saying before a large audience, "I do the same procedure on every patient because aging is always consistent. I don't try to tailor it to any one person." I believe operating this way is dangerous and unfair to his patients. His arrogance may prevent a patient from receiving a better procedure and outcome.

The procedure itself isn't good or bad, but results may be superb when it's used on the right patient and bad if it's used in the wrong patient. Surgeons that do one type of facelift (e.g., deep plane facelift, LifeStyle Lift) market themselves as such, and therefore fit every patient into that technique. This is why some patients look too done. They didn't need all the work that was performed as in a deep plane facelift, or they have very little improvement because they needed more work to be done than the LifeStyle Lift they just underwent.

Your surgeon should have technique versatility to give you what you need not just what they want to do. All noses after surgery don't have to look the same. Facelifts don't need to pull out on the corners of the mouth. All eyebrows don't need to have a semi-circular look. All techniques have advantages, disadvantages, and limitations, which the surgeon should appreciate by fitting the appropriate technique to the appropriate patient.

Protecting Patients from Themselves

Plastic surgeons need to protect patients from themselves. This includes evaluating patients to determine if they're medically stable to undergo the procedure. After a high-profile patient died during an office surgery, it was learned that she'd been turned down by at least two other plastic surgeons because of her medical condition. I'm sure those plastic surgeons were disappointed that they couldn't operate on this patient. But they did the right thing by putting her health above everything else. Unfortunately, someone else didn't.

Longer and more extensive procedures are popular today, but they carry with them higher serious potential risks and complications. One example of this new type of extensive procedure is the "Mommy Makeover." This surgery corrects post-pregnancy problems, including sagging breasts, abdominal protrusion and stretch marks, and weight gain. The surgery typically involves breast augmentation, breast lifts, liposuction, and a tummy tuck.

Other services include the "Large Volume Liposuction," where hours are spent removing fat from many body areas and the "Blue Plate Special," focusing on rejuvenation surgery for the forehead, eyes, and face. The advantage for the patient is having all the work performed under one anesthesia, a cost reduction for multiple procedures, a one-time absence from work, and a single recovery.

But sometimes the risks for the patient outweigh those benefits. *Surgeons should protect their patient from anesthetic complications as well.* The incidence of anesthetic complications increases after five hours of surgery and include heart problems, blood clots, pneumonia, and infection. Even after three hours, increased bleeding and swelling may make performing the surgery more difficult. I have foregone performing a tummy tuck on multiple occasions because the preceding hysterectomy was taking an extended time, putting the patient at a higher anesthetic risk. Here in St. Louis, the anesthesia providers stopped a "Blue Plate Special" procedure by another surgeon at seven o'clock in the evening that had started at seven in the morning. The case was originally scheduled for six hours. The anesthesia staff asked the surgeon to admit the patient for overnight observation. The patient's surgery resumed at seven the next morning and the extensive facelift procedure was completed by noon. By then, the patient had been under 17 hours of general anesthesia. This placed the patient at an unnecessarily greater risk of complications or even death for a purely elective procedure.

Surgery is intense and requires constant concentration to prevent mistakes. Surgeons who believe that they do just as well ten hours into a procedure as they do three hours into the surgery are kidding themself and misleading the patient. It's the surgeon's responsibility to ensure they aren't placing the patient at an increased risk by undergoing the more extensive procedure. It may be better to perform two shorter procedures with two short recoveries than one long surgery with increased risks, a subsequent long recovery, and a greater potential for complications.

The Facility Matters

Joan Rivers may still be alive if her procedure had been performed in a more appropriate outpatient facility. Although it may be more expensive, operating in a quality facility assures adequate staff, medications, and resuscitation equipment.

One of my patients had a cardiac arrest when I was placing a dressing on after a three-hour face- and neck lift. Since I work in a tertiary care center, there were six anesthesiologists in the room immediately and 20 minutes later, my interventional cardiologist friend had placed a stent in one of her heart vessels. If her surgery had been performed at a less equipped surgical facility, 20 minutes later, we would still have been waiting for an ambulance to arrive.

A 2015 report analyzing cosmetic surgery in California revealed that only 16 percent of the over 600 facilities treating over 150,000 patients were accredited facilities.[43] An accredited surgical facility must meet certain minimum standards to obtain and maintain its accreditation. Facility certification requires commitment and money. Nonaccredited facilities don't have to report complications or even deaths to the state medical board for oversite. Besides the Joint Commission to accredit hospitals, two other accreditation organizations exist:

- Accreditation Association for Ambulatory Health Care (AAAHC)
- American Association for Accreditation of Ambulatory Surgical Facilities (AAAASF)

Every year, board-certified plastic surgeons belonging to the ASPS and ASAPS must sign a statement that they'll operate only in accredited surgical facilities. This is important for patient safety. This is also why much of the bad plastic surgery that's performed is in nonaccredited facilities such a hotel rooms, bedrooms, providers' offices, and basements.

I prefer operating in a large hospital with every possible amenity available to care for a patient, especially in a life-threatening situation.

Chapter 14
Complications, Poor Results, or Botched Plastic Surgery

- - - - - - - - - - -

I t is important to distinguish between a complication, a poor result, and really botched surgery. Although not anticipated, complications can arise with any surgical procedure. A poor result can occur if more is expected than what can actually be done. Really botched plastic surgery can occur when patients forego their due diligence.

Complications

Complications are not anticipated but they can and do occur. Dana, whom you met in Chapter 5, had major complications after reconstructive breast surgery done by another surgeon. Instead of using traditional breast implants, her surgeon convinced her to utilize her lower abdominal tissue to reconstruct new breasts. However, after a lengthy, 17-hour surgery, she had complications that required another 10-hour surgery five days later.

After that surgery, there was extensive necrosis and tissue loss in each new "breast," at which point she came to me. She required multiple surgeries over the next few months to correct the problems. She told me that if she had been appropriately informed prior to surgery that the complications could be so severe, she would never have done the surgery. Five

202 | EXPOSING BAD PLASTIC SURGERY

years after her original reconstruction attempt, I completed an implant reconstruction to replace both breasts.

Potential complications are inherent in *any* procedure, including cosmetic, and many of these complications result from the provider's inexperience or lack of knowledge. IPL exposures and laser procedures run the risk of creating dark or white skin patches and skin burns if used inappropriately. Hair loss can also be considered a complication if a light laser is used to correct pigment problems on a male face. Skin rejuvenation with RF technology potentially exposes the skin to a risk of burns if the energy is not appropriately dissipated. Ultrasonic therapies will make the skin and tissue feel funny or "doughy."

There's a small chance of a skin infection at a needle puncture site with every injection. That doesn't sound very likely to occur but if you multiply this risk per injection by the number of injections over the years of using neuromodulators and fillers, it's highly probable that an infection will occur at some point. Sometimes the infection develops deep within the injected material under the skin. This kind of infection should be treated with an anti-inflammatory, antibiotics, or removal of the material and should not be ignored.

The complication rate is higher if the procedure is performed by ancillary staff. In medical spas, the staff is usually educated by the equipment manufacturer, and physician supervision rarely is present onsite. Ancillary personnel are rarely qualified to deal with complications.

Complications still occur even by experienced surgeons. These include but aren't limited to infection, bleeding, scarring, and extended recovery time for healing issues. A trained surgeon is always thinking about and maintaining sterile technique, but a less-qualified provider or a non-surgeon may not fully understand the absolute need for sterility. Lax sterility procedures result in higher infection rates.

Some operations have complications inherent to the procedure. In facial surgery, the nerves for both feeling and motion may be traumatized temporarily but rarely permanently injured. I was asked to defend a local plastic surgeon in a case involving a facial nerve injury after a facelift. The photographs taken by her family two weeks after surgery were devastating to the surgeon's defense as they showed the nerve going to the muscles of her right face had suffered a severe major nerve injury similar to a severe Bell's palsy. She never returned to the surgeon so there were no later pictures to evaluate. I asked her attorney for new pictures but they weren't forthcoming. Six months later, the case was dropped. The patient's attorney called me to tell me, as I expected, that the injury had completely resolved and he could no longer justify the case against the surgeon. Even my patients have complications at times. In one instance, a patient had an eyebrow drop down because of a nerve injury during a facelift surgery. I was able to reassure the patient that the nerve would function again because I knew the only reason the nerve wasn't working was because of the pull of the "lift" and the subsequent temporary traction injury on the nerve. Indeed, it was fully functional six weeks after her surgery.

Other surgeries can have more frequent complications. Contour irregularities after liposuction occur 10 to 20 percent of the time. Complications after extremity lifts approach 40 percent.[44] Ten to 40 percent of breast implant patients may require reoperation.[45] I typically inform my breast augmentation patients that they'll likely undergo at least one other surgery for their implants during their lifetime.

An experienced plastic surgeon learns how to care for complications during a certified plastic surgery training program in reconstructive and burn surgery. These trainees learn how to take injured tissue and structures and make them look normal again. They also develop these skills because they often have to care for complications when patients come to them for help after having surgery with less-qualified providers in the community.

A board-certified plastic surgeon also has a network of surgeons they may turn to for help. For example, a plastic surgeon in Houston had a significant complication after breast reduction surgery. When the patient came to St. Louis ten days later to care for an ailing parent, the Houston plastic surgeon called me to help care for his patient. I was happy to help both the patient and the plastic surgeon. In another example, I was able to call plastic surgeons around the country to ask their advice regarding inflamed stretch marks occurring after breast augmentation. Through my connections, I learned that these could be resolved using IPL phototherapy.

Non-board-certified surgeons don't have this advantage. I believe the complication rates are higher and the complications more severe when non-board-certified "plastic surgeons" perform surgery. But there's no centralized reporting mechanism of complications for these physicians practicing outside of their certified scope of practice.

I've seen many patients with extreme complications after their provider has told them to "find a plastic surgeon to take care of the problem." These patients are stunned and bewildered because they thought their provider *was* a plastic surgeon.

I find it hard to understand the hubris some physicians possess to do surgical procedures they aren't qualified to do. A patient had three skin cancers removed on his forehead by a provider who advertised as a plastic surgeon. The patient was left with three large holes in his forehead that the "plastic surgeon" couldn't pull together. The patient was advised to "quickly find a plastic surgeon" that Friday afternoon. The patient knew me because I'd previously performed eyelid surgery and a facelift on his wife. She called the office and we stayed late into the night to close her husband's large, open wounds. It's always better to have an established relationship with a board-certified plastic surgeon prior to a complication.

Disappointed Expectations

Celebrate the improvement and don't dwell on what is "wrong."

A poor result may be otherwise acceptable but not exactly what you wanted. You may have also thought that you'd obtain something different from the procedure. The feeling of not meeting plastic surgery goals is commonly referred to as "disappointed expectations." The patient must reassess if their anticipated result was actually obtainable based on preoperative reality. The "expected" result may have been unobtainable regardless of who did the procedure.

After surgical procedures, you should expect significant improvements within the limitations present before surgery. If you have a thick nasal tip, you shouldn't expect a well-defined tip after nasal surgery because thinning the tip too much may cause a horrible result. A thick preoperative neck will never look like the thin neck of a one-hundred-pound woman. The augmentation of uneven breasts will rarely result in absolute symmetry. As an older plastic surgeon told me, "It's possible to make sisters but almost impossible to create twins." A patient undergoing a tummy tuck after multiple births shouldn't expect the abdominal wall of a 22-year-old woman who's never had children. A middle-aged woman undergoing liposuction shouldn't expect to look like a 24-old after the procedure.

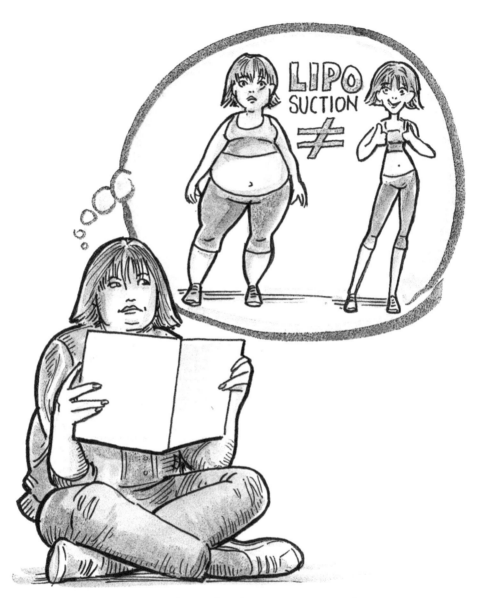

Sometimes a poor result can be the consequence of a poor procedure selection. Frances, my patient mentioned earlier in the book, falls into this category even though she thought she was doing everything right. You can't expect a 90 percent improvement if you choose a noninvasive procedure that can only provide a 30 percent improvement at best. Pushing a noninvasive laser procedure to simulate surgical results may result in an unnatural, waxy look to the skin without the natural brown or red color and loss of the skin's soft texture. Too much neuromodulator in the wrong places could leave you "frozen."

If the provider you selected only performs less-invasive procedures, you may end up with an injected, overfilled face when you also needed tightening of sagging skin only a facelift can provide. A qualified surgeon can more appropriately remove loose, sagging skin and minimally enhance the supporting structures with filler. A natural look that doesn't look "done" requires a multi-technique approach appropriately addressing each problem. But, if the surgeon only performs one type of facelift, and you need more or something different, you won't be happy with your less-than-ideal result if the surgeon performs his "usual" on you.

Patient actions after surgery can also create a poor result. Poor patient compliance to postoperative instructions may detract from a good surgical procedure. Some patients just won't follow appropriate postoperative instructions supplied by their surgeon or get "confused" because they read something online that better suits what they want to do. The patient referenced earlier in the book who, against our specific instructions not to scratch or peel off the shedding skin after her chemical peel, picked off all the skin because she said it itched. Her noncompliance has left her with permanent scarring.

A surgeon has a specific postoperative routine, which the surgeon feels gives the best result. The patient should adhere to the experienced professional's routine. I had a patient who underwent a neck lift. The next day, she removed the supportive neck garment because it interfered with her social life. She went golfing on the second postoperative day although she'd been instructed not to bend over for the first week after surgery. Because the neck skin wasn't supported and couldn't adhere to the underlying muscles, the neck skin became loose and floppy. Correction required another surgery and more "appropriate" postoperative care and restrictions.

Beth, another patient, also exhibited a poor result because of her actions after surgery. A weight gain of 75 pounds after her "mommy makeover" surgery resulted in horrible contour deformities, cancer confusion, and an unhappy patient. She told me she noticed some of these problems after an initial weight gain of 20 pounds but confessed that she thought she could continue and just have the surgery all redone. She didn't like my recommendation to lose weight even though we gave a number of references to help her.

Bad scars are frequently referred to as plastic surgery gone badly. How often have you seen headlines suggesting that a patient has been left with "Frankenstein scars" and has been scarred forever by bad plastic surgery? Bad scars in plastic surgery aren't necessarily bad plastic surgery but only a poor outcome that's out of the control of the operating physician. No surgeon wants a bad scar because it's there forever. The scar becomes an outward symbol of the work performed by that surgeon.

Botched Plastic Surgery

Gloria and Jeanne surely had what I consider to be "botched plastic surgery" by less than skilled providers. Gloria had no idea about the true qualifications of the surgeon who operated on her in Mexico. She just wanted it done cheaply in a place she could vacation afterwards. She was left with major complications and botched outcomes on every area of her body that was operated on. Jeanne went to a less-than-qualified physician initially who overestimated her skin's ability to shrink, leaving her with loose, hanging, inner thigh skin. If the surgeon who operated on her twice had been properly trained, they would have appreciated the fact that this complication can be avoided with appropriate skin removal and a thoughtful placement of stabilizing sutures to prevent opening the perineum.

The bad plastic surgery results pictured in the tabloids are often caused by injectables. The neuromodulators are short lived, and if you look weird, the effects of the neuromodulator will dissipate in a few months. Most fillers are temporary and last six months to five years. The temporary fillers will just go away or can be hurried along by dissolving them with an enzyme that works immediately. Surgical removal of fillers is fraught with contour problems since the filler is embedded in the patient's own tissue. Removal of the filler means removal of the soft tissue, too, leaving an indentation. And one surgery may not be enough to remove all the filler. For years, a patient from Columbia came to me for surgery twice a year to remove silicone that had been injected into her face in her home country 15 years earlier.

Fat injections pose a significant potential for complications since there are no good remedies for less-than-ideal results. Faces overfilled with fat can potentially have the fat dissolved with chemicals or removed with liposuction, but it is seldom an ideal result.

The experienced, board-certified plastic surgeon will understand the nuances of a surgical procedure and will be able to help if results are botched. They gain most of their experience dealing with complications of burns, healing wounds, and reconstructing cancer defects. During their training, plastic surgeons learn how to fix things and put parts back together after they've been deformed or even destroyed. Plastic surgeons gain a lot of their corrective experience taking care of botched plastic surgery from other providers. Training programs in plastic surgery are typically tertiary care referral centers for revision surgeries, and therefore, plastic surgeons in their training see and learn a lot about correcting bad outcomes. *No other provider has this experience to correct the defects resulting from bad plastic surgery.*

Remember, though, corrective surgery by a competent plastic surgeon will probably cost more than if you'd had the initial surgery performed by that surgeon. More time and expertise are required to correct bad surgery than having it done correctly the first time.

Chapter 15
How to Avoid Bad Plastic Surgery

- - - - - - - - - - - -

Now that you have some ideas about why there's so much bad plastic surgery, it's time to give you tips and pointers on how you can avoid it. Like a bad tattoo, I don't want you to regret your surgical or nonsurgical interventions every time you look in the mirror. And I know you don't want to show up to your high school or college reunion and hear everyone gasp.

Seek the Best; Find the Best; Expect the Best

This is probably the most concise advice I can give to a patient contemplating plastic surgery or injectable therapies. Be an *active participant* in selecting the professional to whom you're entrusting your face and body. Advocate for yourself because you have the most at stake and the greatest desire for the best result.

In the following pages, you'll be given a set of 13 suggestions to use before, during, and after your surgery. These are meant to guide you to a successful result, one that you'll be happy about having it done with a surgeon who was right for you.

You must be a discerning consumer when considering plastic surgery. As consumers, we may spend more time and research picking out a new car than we spend choosing our plastic surgeon. We also may spend less money on our plastic surgeon than on a car that we may use only five to seven years. In contrast to a new car, surgical improvement lasts for a lifetime. With good plastic surgery, you look good even without being in your new car. It just doesn't make sense to bargain shop on something you and others will see every day and for the rest of your life—you!

Even before starting your research, reflect on why you want to proceed with a surgery that will change your appearance. Make sure that you're doing it for yourself. Having a facelift won't save your marriage. Having a breast augmentation won't stop a boyfriend's eyes from wandering. Having nasal surgery won't get you elected as prom queen. Don't do it because of pressure from a partner, a friend, or your family. The only way you'll be happy with your result is if you are, first and foremost, doing it only for *yourself* and making your decision based upon what a surgeon or procedure can do particularly for *you*.

1. Be Sure You Know What It Is That Bothers You.

Be sure you know what you want prior to any consultation with a provider. Take time to review your desires, and don't make hasty decisions. Patients tend to be the happiest when they know exactly what they want to achieve. Many of my patients tell me they had been researching and thinking about having a procedure done for years.

A vague dislike of your face or body isn't helpful to your surgeon. A woman came to me to discuss her "face issues." She'd consulted at least two other plastic surgeons before our initial visit. Yet, when I asked her what bothered her most, she responded, "I don't really know. You're the expert." She apparently wanted *me* to tell her what was wrong with her face! I did what I could, which meant a thorough analysis of her face with her looking in the mirror. When I finished, she still couldn't put together a list of priorities for herself. With a lack of definitive ideas about what she thinks is wrong, there's little chance that any surgeon would make her happy.

2. Be Certain of the Result You Want.

As has been discussed in previous chapters, different procedures provide different results. Noninvasive or less-invasive procedures can't provide the same result as surgery. Nonsurgical procedures make small changes and subtle improvements. But nonsurgical results are variable with improvement ranging from 10 to 15 percent and they last only a few years at best. Lasers, RF, ultrasound, freezing, heating, and injectables should be considered if you're concerned about costs, downtime, and risks—and will accept subtle improvements. No machine or injectable exists that will give you a 50 percent improvement with a couple of days of downtime. Nonsurgical treatments often need to be repeated, and the total cost of these may approach the cost of surgery itself. Be wary of practitioners pushing less-invasive procedures saying they can match the dramatic results of surgery. They push these procedures because they aren't qualified to perform surgical interventions.

The bottom line is that, at best, minimally invasive rejuvenation offers only modest improvements to the patient. This is an example of publicity and marketing overpromising the reality and validity of scientific data. The perfect or ideal technology for producing results that match expectations, delivers on promises, and mimics surgery hasn't yet arrived on the market.

Surgery should be considered if you're looking for an 80 percent improvement and can afford a couple of weeks of downtime. Surgery is more predictable, achieves significant improvements, and lasts 10 to 15 years. Many surgical patients have a procedure and then continue along the normal aging process. This is referred to as "daylight savings time surgery" because these patients continue to age but their "clock" has been set back. If you go the surgical route, you'll have to accept that there will be more initial expense, the use of general anesthesia, and necessary downtime, probably calculated in weeks, to recover after the procedure.

If you decide against undergoing a surgical procedure because of general anesthesia and an extended recovery and, instead, go the nonsurgical route, you may be left very unhappy. Remember that the correct procedure, with a two- to three-week recovery, will provide a more dramatic and long-lasting improvement than 30 minutes under a laser.

Because I have a surgeon's mentality, I believe more in aesthetic surgery than aesthetic medicine. I have seen the results of these newer technologies in patients who end up in my office and I often cannot distinguish the post-procedure appearance from a pre-procedure photograph. Our patient Frances who presented with a black garage bag full of "gadgets, gizmos, and potions" was one such patient. At best, minimally invasive rejuvenation devices offer only modest benefits and the ideal technology for delivering the results the patient expects has yet to be available in the present marketplace. Almost all new technologies promote and promise increased collagen production, but this means increased damage to the soft tissues. I have operated on many patients who have been dissatisfied with the results of these noninvasive technologies and I find the treated tissue edematous (filled with fluid) and firm without natural elastic properties. If you, as a patient, are willing to commit to surgery, your final result will be more satisfying and longer lasting. After years of decreasing surgical numbers because of noninvasive technology, facelift surgery has increased in the last four years. More patients just want to have surgery, get it over, and move on rather than repeating the noninvasive treatments again and again and then again with the next "latest and greatest new technology" promoted by the manufacturers.

Patients tend to be the happiest when they know what they want to change, attain, and achieve. They understand the limitations of nonsurgical intervention and that it may end up costing as much as surgery. If you decide on surgery, be prepared for the time needed for recovery and the physical change. Just know that this physical change will be only one aspect of "feeling good about yourself."

3. Do Your Research.

Research the procedure as well as the surgeon prior to your consultation. Patients often spend more time researching investment choices, home, and car purchases, or arranging their next vacation than researching a procedure or the person who could permanently alter their looks.

Research the Procedure

Research the procedure before making your decision, but be sure it's accurate and trustworthy. Be generally skeptical of information you find on the internet. Select reputable sources to learn from such as peer-reviewed medical literature and medical journals. Wikipedia articles aren't a good substitute for well-sourced medical literature and may contain wrong information. News sites may be more accurate. Google has attempted to improve its accuracy of medical search results by fact-checking and displaying information verified by physicians at Google and the Mayo Clinic. Sponsored sites, which pay premiums to be listed first, are rarely accurate. These sponsored sites are selling a product or service and are less concerned about accuracy in information.

While many legitimate websites have information about surgical procedures, much of this information falls into the "difficult" to read or comprehend categories unless you're in a medical profession.

Better sites for information gathering include academic institutional sites (e.g., Cleveland Clinic, Mayo Clinic, Johns Hopkins, etc.) and plastic surgery society sites such as the American Society of Plastic Surgery (www.plasticsurgery.org) and the American Society of Aesthetic Plastic Surgery (www.surgery.org). These plastic surgery society sites give excellent descriptions of the surgical procedures and provide basic information on member surgeons.

Don't request a specific operation or treatment because of an advertisement or a blog post. You may not be a good candidate for that specific procedure. Your surgeon should have technique versatility and be your best resource for information. Your result is more dependent on who performs the operation and much less on the technique that's used. Please listen carefully to the doctor who's spent many years training in order to appropriately advise you. Qualified surgeons can and will make appropriate technique recommendations for you as an individual.

Research Your Potential Physicians

Patients today often use the internet as their source of choice to find their plastic surgeon, and many assume that if a plastic surgeon shows up on the first page of a Google search, they must be good. Unfortunately, skill as a surgeon isn't how Google ranks plastic surgeons. A first-page ranking only means the physician has optimized their website using SEO and is active on multiple social media accounts. In other words, they have a big online presence. But that presence says nothing about their ability to do their work well. Believing a first-page ranking on Google is more important than a physician's schooling, experience, expertise, ability, and results is a big mistake.

Seek physicians with years of experience or a physician with a particular expertise. Again, your final result is more related to the surgeon you choose than the technique chosen. The surgeon you select should tailor the procedure to your concerns. Choose your surgeon by their credentials. It's important that they have an excellent reputation and practice at highly credentialed facilities. Make sure you know which specialty certifies your surgeon and if that specialty is legitimate and recognized by the ABMS. You can check their board certification at www.ABMS.org or www.CertificationMatters.org. Also, as noted above, visit the plastic surgery societies' websites to search for board-certified members (www.plasticsurgery.org and www.surgery.org).

Don't fall victim to the many pretenders out there such as the surgical assistant who posed as a plastic surgeon and ran his own cosmetic surgery clinic in Denver, Colorado, for over 18 months.[46] He used titles such as "Doctor" and "Plastic Surgeon" and administered medications and wrote prescriptions. He advertised that he performed facelifts, nasal surgery, breast augmentation, liposuction, and tummy tucks. He had five out of five-star ratings on numerous rating sites. The procedures were performed in his clinic with no general anesthesia and only local anesthesia and Valium. He was eventually charged with ten felonies including criminal impersonation, illegally practicing medicine, sexual abuse, child abuse, and second-degree assault. According to the arrest affidavit, he was arrested in his cosmetic surgery clinic while performing an "invasive surgical procedure," and the scalpel was taken from him as an offending weapon.

Always be skeptical of medical treatment by people not licensed to be medical professionals.

4. Get Recommendations for Your Surgery from People You Trust.

I'm reminded of an Alfred Hitchcock movie where an assessment of advertising was given by the main character: "In the world of advertising, there is no such thing as a lie. There is only expedient exaggeration."[47]

Advertising serves a useful purpose, but not, perhaps, when you're searching for a plastic surgeon. If a surgeon is trying to attract you to their office by promoting the next greatest thing or by saying they're the greatest, be cautious. They may be a "one-trick pony," a doctor who can only do one type of procedure. And, honestly, if you have to say you're great, you probably aren't.

Remember my earlier warnings of preoperative and postoperative photographs?

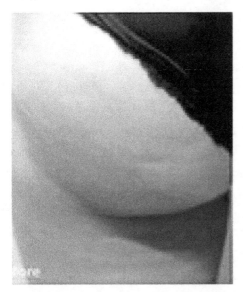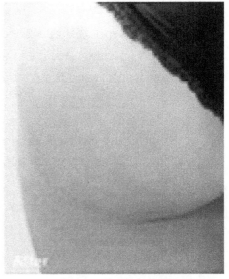

An advertisement for an external skin tightening machine to also reduce cellulite utilizes overhead lighting for the pre-procedure picture...note the shadow in her inner buttock fold (left) and direct lighting for the picture showing the "result" (right). The photographs were probably taken within seconds of each other as the patient is wearing the exact same undergarment with the same ruffles at the exact same angle across her buttock mound.

These photos will represent only their best results and may even have been purchased. If a photo only shows their "fabulous result," it may be prudent to assume these "postoperative" photographs could be models who haven't been surgery patients of the advertised surgeon. A plastic surgeon was disciplined after his advertisement had a picture of a Ferrari and a "patient" under the headline of "Car by Ferrari…Body by Dr. Smith." Unfortunately, Dr. Smith never operated on the "patient"/model.

Even though board-certified plastic surgeons are required to identify a model as such, some don't. In a twist of irony, a postoperative patient of mine became a paid model for another plastic surgeon's advertisement in St. Louis. The surgeon selected her photos to demonstrate one of "his results" and didn't identify her as a paid model. There was really nothing I could do about the advertisement, as it was done under the guise of "business."

Look with skepticism at every advertisement you see, and watch out for intended vagueness. Accuracy and clarity will convey the appropriate message and being vague is a cover-up. A multi-physician plastic surgery group in the Midwest advertises: "Our physicians have received countless prestigious awards…" Which should right away make you ask: what physicians in this group received these awards? If one physician received these "awards," don't I want to go to that physician? I can count to at least one thousand; therefore, is "countless awards" more than a thousand? What are the "prestigious" awards these physicians have received? Is it a "parent of the year" award and nothing to do with medicine? If they were really "prestigious awards" that may be recognized by the public, would it not be appropriate to list these "awards" so that the reader may be impressed?

Always look for precision in advertisements. I would love to see a disclaimer required at the bottom of every plastic surgery advertisement similar to what advertisements for attorneys in Missouri must state: "The choice of a lawyer is an important decision and should not be based solely upon advertisement."

The same holds true when choosing your plastic surgeon.

Internet Advertising

Nowadays, most advertising for plastic surgeons is done on the internet. Unfortunately, the internet is a great equalizer. Everyone is *the best* and *the greatest* on their website. Some even describe themselves as *unparalleled* or *peerless*. Understand that physician websites are electronic marketing sites that exist with no oversight from a higher authority. Marketers know what catches the public eye and exploit this knowledge. Vague superlatives are overused and misused on these websites. Below are a few of these along with what they may actually mean:

What the Website Says	What the Words Really Mean
Internationally known	Has a sister living in England
Nationally renowned	Belongs to a national organization
Highly sought	By marketing companies
Doctor's doctor	Stitched a finger laceration on another physician
Locally respected	By their church community
Locally renowned	By their neighborhood

Sometimes you'll see the word "institute" on a website. What that usually means is an organization created for a particular purpose. The impression the website is going for is of a medical institute, a group of physicians academically challenged to deliver the best. Unfortunately, more common than not, "institute" is used to describe a solo practitioner performing plastic surgery as their particular purpose and nothing more.

Remember, the premium listings at the top of an internet search for plastic surgery or "breast augmentation in (your city)" are paid listings. The advertising entity is charged per "hit" by the research engine. This "pay per click" advertising is a legitimate way of buying yourself to the top of an internet search. These premium listings have nothing to do with a surgeon's expertise or reputation, and they may not even be advertisements for board-certified plastic surgeons. Just remember, premium listings are simply paid advertisements that anyone can purchase.

Rating Websites

These sites have been extensively discussed in previous chapters, most notably Chapter 6. Suffice it to say, rating websites should rarely *impact* your decision when choosing your surgeon because they don't rate the things that are important, like achieving a good result after surgery. Instead, ratings sites focus on areas that have little to no impact on results (e.g., office décor, phone response time, etc.). Yet, time after time, physicians will achieve a five out of five rating, giving these minor qualities outsized importance. A physician is more likely to receive a negative review for bad service than for bad medicine.

Please remember, a physician's online reputation is an incomplete and unbalanced representation of that physician's practice. It doesn't adequately address the plastic surgeon's knowledge, operative skills, diagnostic skills, communication skills, or surgical outcomes. Besides, there's no data to suggest that improved surgical outcomes correlate with patient satisfaction ratings.

Surgeons have tried, without success, to make ratings sites take down inappropriate ratings and even downright lies. But physician rating sites are felt to be "opinion sites" by the courts, where people can voice an opinion. The courts ruled that readers should realize these are one person's opinion and free speech rights apply even if the statements are proven false. I hope everyone who reads internet reviews understands the sites are opinions and not necessarily factual.

What may be more eye opening than an online rating site review are the results of a patient satisfaction survey conducted in 2018.[48] Thirty-seven thousand patients who underwent surgery by over seven hundred plastic surgeons provided answers to a number of questions regarding patient satisfaction after their plastic surgery. The researchers found that satisfaction is most affected by surgeon-related factors and not service issues. The strongest factors that resulted in satisfied patients were 1) the patient's level of confidence in the surgeon as developed through communication and reputation, 2) the surgeon's concern for the patient's questions and worries, 3) the surgeon taking time to address patient's concerns and answering questions, and 4) including the patient in the decision-making process. Choose your plastic surgeon based on these four factors and you'll more likely get a great result.

Recommendations the Old-Fashioned Way

Instead of relying on the internet, I recommend you use the tried-and-true way of finding your plastic surgeon by asking for references from trusted advisors. These people include your physician, close friends, and previous patients of that surgeon. Physicians tend to hear "the word on the street" about plastic surgeons and also see the results.

If your obstetrics and gynecology physician suggest you go to a particular plastic surgeon for a breast augmentation, their recommendation is probably reliable because they see so many post-augmentation patients during well-patient exams. I performed breast augmentations on five close friends who walked together every morning. It all started when an ob–gyn physician recommended the first woman to me.

I have one warning to keep in mind when you ask physicians for recommendations. Some physicians refer patients to plastic surgeons who are in their social circles. They sometimes overlook a bad reputation to send the patient to their friend. Although not acceptable in medicine, some poorly qualified surgeons even offer a finder's fee to another physician for a referral.

If you're seeking a breast augmentation, another good source are mammogram technologists. They see a lot of breasts every day and typically don't have an established friendship with one plastic surgeon.

Previous plastic surgery patients, who may also be your good friends, are a great recommendation source. I'm always amazed at how open plastic surgery patients are to discuss their surgery with someone they may not know well. Some even show off their results. I reconstructed three sisters after each had breast cancer surgery, but only the first one lived in

St. Louis. A friend of the first sister had breast reconstruction performed by me for breast cancer and recommended my practice. Another St. Louis patient on whom I'd performed a facelift referred her friend in Singapore to me for that procedure. Friends and acquaintances, if they're satisfied with their results, will happily refer others to their surgeon.

Nurses are also good a source for recommendations. They are a witness to the physician's personality, skills, and outcomes. An operating room nurse may steer you clear of a surgeon who just Googled "how to do a facelift" on the computer in the operating room. (Yes, that happened at our hospital.) Nurses also see complications because these patients usually need to be admitted to the hospital for ongoing treatment. Remember Dana? She was in the intensive care unit of a local teaching hospital after her two botched breast reconstructions. She asked every nurse in the intensive care unit who they'd go to if they had this complication. When she was stable enough, she signed herself out against medical advice and showed up in my office on her way home.

Don't seek advice about plastic surgery from a plastic surgeon in social circles or at parties. A good surgeon should never give a medical assessment based on the limited information gathered at a dinner or a party. If you like the surgeon after you meet them at a social function, it's best to set up an appointment to see them.

Thankfully, most patients don't use social media to select their plastic surgeon. The aforementioned satisfaction study asked patients what information they considered before making their choice of plastic surgeon.[49] Over 40 percent considered the reputation of the surgeon the most important. Thirty-five percent were recommended to their surgeon by a previous patient and less than 20 percent considered the surgeon's website to be important. Only 5 percent considered social media in their selection. Of the small percentage of patients who even looked at social media, over 50 percent felt it didn't help very much but confirmed what they already knew. Some felt that it helped their decision to steer clear of a surgeon.

Solid facts and the physician's background are more important than superlative interpretations. Do your homework. Ask your other physicians, listen to a previous patient's recommendations, review the surgeon's academic training, and assess the surgeon's reputation based on many years of good results. Qualifications matter. Remember, you're buying the doctor and their expertise first. The procedure is secondary.

5. Don't Rely Only on a Virtual Consult.

Part of an appropriate evaluation of a patient is actually touching the tissue and the skin to feel if these can be surgically manipulated. An appropriate physical exam will determine whether or not the tissues can be elevated, stretched, or repositioned and if the anticipated result can be accomplished.

A touch will tell you more about the condition of the tissue than looking at it in a picture. Sometimes tugging on the eyebrows will convince you that a brow lift will cause horrible dry eye problems because the brow lift will prevent the eyelids from completely closing, thereby exposing the cornea. Pulling the lower eyelid away from the eye globe will show a lower eyelid laxity that may result in a "hound dog" droop if lower eyelid surgery is performed. Pushing up on the cheek may disclose a deep tissue tethering that will prevent a full deep tissue release, thus preventing the ability to adequately perform a cheek lift. Pressing on the nasal tip may reveal lack of structural support or thickened skin that will obscure any fine cartilage work performed underneath the tip. None of these things can be even guessed at by looking at a photograph or a video image.

However, some providers perform patient evaluations using virtual technology anyway. These offices accept your electronically transmitted photographs to evaluate you as a candidate for potential surgery. After emailing or uploading your photographs, you'll begin a back-and-forth discussion online with the office to determine your eligibility for the procedure or surgery. For in-person visits, some offices take pictures before any evaluation starts. These pictures are then printed and given to the provider before they enter the patient's room. I hesitate to call it an exam room because often a true exam is never performed. Many patients have told me that oftentimes the provider completes the history by asking the concerns of the patient and then "evaluates" the patient by using the photographs to point out areas that need attention. The provider never touches the patient.

A twenty-four-year-old patient told me that her "evaluation" for breast augmentation at another provider's office consisted having photos taken of her breasts and a discussion with the provider who, using editing software, showed her what her results would look like. No one ever touched her breasts during this evaluation. During my physical examination, a small mass was found in her right breast. A biopsy confirmed it was breast cancer. Instead of breast augmentation surgery, she underwent the appropriate breast cancer treatment.

The physical exam, actually touching the tissue, is an important part of a patient's examination prior to a procedure or surgery. As an old general surgeon once taught me, "The hands will reveal what the eyes may not perceive."

6. Call the Surgeon's Office.

Avoid communicating with the office only online. Don't make your appointment through the physician's website. Call the office and speak with the employees. The staff should be pleasant, engaging, and competent. Ask about the physician's specific board certification. Merely asking if the physician is board-certified is too broad. A physician may be board-certified in General Surgery but not Plastic Surgery. You probably don't want a surgeon who operates mainly on gall bladders doing your tummy tuck or your facelift. Ask specifically in what specialty they're board-certified.

You may want to inquire about an approximate number of cases like yours that the doctor has performed. Be suspect if the answer is five thousand or a similar large number. One physician in St. Louis advertised that he has performed over twenty thousand procedures. Sounds impressive until you do the math. If he's done that many, it means he's spent six years doing ten procedures every day (three hundred and sixty-five days a year), or twelve years doing five procedures every day, or twenty years of doing four procedures every weekday without vacations or holidays. Likely? I think not.

When inquiring about price, expect a range of cost because the staff can't tell over the phone what may make your surgery different. Liposuction is a good example of this. You should expect a range of costs because the staff can't tell how many areas need to be addressed or the time required to achieve the result. Both of these issues will have a bearing on cost. It's best to wait until your consultation to ask about costs. Some offices give low prices over the phone to get you in the door and then give you the real costs in the office.

7. Don't Bargain Shop.

Don't spend four thousand dollars on a Yugo and expect the looks and performance of a Ferrari around two hundred fifty thousand). I can't overstate this: Now isn't the time to bargain shop. Don't buy "knockoff plastic surgery," and don't decide who will perform your procedure based on money. Remember that discounted plastic surgery may actually cost more. Rock-bottom advertised rates may not include the hidden costs of the operating room, implants, anesthesia, or injectable material. On top of that, it may compromise the quality of the materials and workmanship and your safety. Many clinic or office settings lack basic equipment such as ventilators and defibrillators. Their "visiting" anesthesiologist leaves the building before you do.

Don't forfeit standards for price, as the results often don't satisfy the expectations. The money is worth it for the extra quality and safety of going to an appropriate physician at an appropriately certified facility. Many cheaper noncertified surgery facilities make money by putting large numbers of patients rapidly through the facility. With low-cost margins, they may have to cut costs by using inexperienced staff, second-rate supplies, or inadequate anesthesia staff or monitoring. Remember, noncertified facilities often lack appropriate oversight and supervision.

Joan Rivers was a great ambassador for plastic surgery. She was never shy about her plastic surgery and spoke of her procedures often. But she succumbed to a complication during a procedure that may have been avoided if she would've listened to her own advice.

Multiple times in her cosmetic surgery advice book entitled *Men Sre Stupid…and They Like Big Boobs*, she warns of death as a possible complication and how to avoid it:

- "The risk is all but nil…since you will be operated on in an accredited facility by a board-certified plastic surgeon with a board-certified anesthesiologist."
- "If you use a board-certified doctor and have the procedure done in an accredited facility, your chances of dying are slim to none."
- "Make sure the facility is equipped with all the necessary lifesaving apparatus."[50]

Joan Rivers underwent a procedure on her vocal cords in an outpatient endoscopy facility poorly equipped to handle an unintended (though possible) airway complication. By the time professionally trained emergency medical technician (EMT) staff arrived at the facility, it was too late. Joan Rivers died because she had surgery at a facility that was not equipped with the necessary lifesaving equipment/drugs and a well-trained staff as espoused in her own book.

A patient who came to me for revision surgery said that after her first surgery in an office operating room, she was placed into a taxi still sedated. The physician's staff complained in front of the cab driver and the patient that it was late and they were missing dinner. The cabbie deposited her in the foyer of her apartment building where her friend later found her propped up against the marble wall and nearly incoherent. The physician's office never called the friend to let her know that the patient was ready to be picked up.

As with this patient, you may later incur the costs of revising or correcting botched plastic surgery, and this revision work will be expensive. I've had many patients tell my staff that the revision surgery cost more than their initial surgery. This is usually true since correcting bad results is more complicated and takes longer than the initial surgery.

If you can't afford your surgery now, put it off until you can. You'll have to look at yourself every day after the surgery; it's best to wait and invest the money and time it will take to get the result you want. You may be able to work out financing with the surgeon's office either in-house or through an outside financial institution. These financing options allow the patient to have the surgery as well as ongoing care and maybe other procedures. Remember that your choice of surgeon and their expertise is critical to the final result and your happiness. If you can't do it *now* with the surgeon of your choice, do it *later* with that surgeon when you are more fiscally stable. As I always say, "You can pay me now or you can pay me *more* later."

8. Consult with Several Different Surgeons.

Most of the patients I see have visited another plastic surgeon before their consultation with me. Some patients have a consultation with me and then come back later after consulting with other surgeons. I encourage a patient who's seeing me for a first consultation to talk with a second physician prior to deciding upon surgery. One patient saw six different surgeons for a breast augmentation consultation before choosing me two years later. She told me that she really wanted to be sure and the time was just not right when I first saw her.

If you walk out of a consultation knowing you want that surgeon to care for you, then by all means continue on with that surgeon. If you don't feel that way, see someone else even if that second consultation costs you. Paying for multiple consultations is money well spent. Many plastic surgeons even offer free consultations.

Remember, you're buying the surgeon and their expertise first and the procedure second.

9. Show Up to Your Consultation with Questions and Concerns.

Good plastic surgery isn't obtained in the operating room alone. You and your physician will become a team, both wanting to achieve a great outcome and a satisfied patient. This is a shared decision, and both patient and physician should take part in deciding what procedure is best. At your initial consultation, the physician should utilize their knowledge, experience, and expertise to decide on an appropriate plan for you. Let the plastic surgeon educate you on the procedure and the recovery. Continue asking questions until everything makes sense *to you*.

Also, the surgeon is evaluating you as much as you are evaluating them. They're deciding whether your concerns are legitimate, if you're a good candidate for the surgery, if you're medically stable, and whether they can give you the result that you desire. Be truthful about medical conditions, as a surgeon won't want to put you at any increased risk for complications. This is elective surgery, and the risks should be minimal. In my training at Johns Hopkins, one patient neglected to tell the surgeon about her heart problems and underwent a facelift. She took her own nitroglycerin tablets the first night after surgery while in the hospital. She didn't tell the nurse that she was having chest pain. She succumbed to heart complications eight days after her elective surgery.

One of my patients didn't think to tell me that six months earlier, her daughter had died of a sudden heart problem while out walking. As I was putting the dressing on after her facelift, she had a severe cardiac arrhythmia. Because I perform my facelifts in our level one trauma rated hospital, she was seen by a cardiologist in the recovery room within 20 minutes and taken to the heart catheterization lab for an interventional procedure. She did well postoperatively. Another patient failed to tell us about a strong family history of blood clots because she believed, appropriately, that I'd pass on her surgery. She had a blood clot in her lungs on the second day after surgery. She survived only because she'd decided to stay in the hospital an extra day.

Go to your consults with written notes to help you remember your questions.

Below are some questions to ask your surgeon:

1. Are you currently licensed by the state and certified in the designated area of surgery?
2. Am I a good candidate?
3. What do you recommend for me and why?
4. Is it different than what you would normally perform?
5. Where do you do the surgery? Is that facility fully accredited?
6. At what hospital can you perform the surgery if I request it?
7. When can I get back to work or my favorite activity?
8. Will you provide me with a written estimate and does it include everything?
9. If there are complications requiring another surgery, what are the policies of the office?

Noncertified providers tend to overpromise and underdeliver. Certified plastic surgeons are taught that it's best to under-promise but over-deliver. Appropriate board certification and hospital accreditation are a validation of the surgeon's competency.

At the end of the initial consultation, many offices ask for a commitment from you to schedule your surgery and put down a deposit before you leave the office. Some even offer a discount if you sign up on that day. Only do this if you are 100 percent comfortable with the surgeon and the office staff. It's probably better if you at least think about it overnight.

One patient came to see me after her initial consultation with another plastic surgery group in town. She was uncomfortable with the consultation and told the patient coordinator that she "wanted to think about it first" when she was asked to schedule the procedure. She showed me monthly mailed solicitations offering a discount if she would "sign up for surgery in the next month." Then the emails started from the patient care coordinator.

Dear Jeanette,

Just wanted to send you a quick email to let you know about our newest special! If you have your cosmetic surgery procedure before March 31st, you will receive 15% off the surgeon's fee for your first procedure and 20% off the surgeon's fee for your second procedure. This can save you hundreds of dollars. So now you can save money and look great for spring. We only have a few surgery times left in March, so please let me know as soon as possible so you may schedule surgery. OR (operating room) times are going fast!

~ Debbie (Patient Coordinator)

After the third email, Jeanette admitted to feeling harassed. This email is a good example of inducing FOMO in prospective patients by suggesting there may no longer be operating room times available and you'll "miss out," thereby giving someone else the opportunity and the result that you want.

So how do you choose the surgeon into whose hands you're placing your appearance and potentially your life? Even before you meet the surgeon, the office staff should be professional, courteous, and knowledgeable. Your surgeon should respect your time, listen carefully and intently to your concerns, and thoroughly explain their recommendations. The surgeon should be approachable to your secondary questions and you should be comfortable with their competence. Finally, you must feel that you'll work well together.

When you select a doctor, you're authorizing that doctor to make decisions for you. Your doctor should be qualified to make medical and surgical decisions on your behalf. Be comfortable with releasing control to that physician. Most nonqualified providers don't have the training or experience to make appropriate decisions for you. This ability only comes with years of training as well as treating actual patients. It can't be taught at a weekend training course.

10. Schedule a Second Consultation.

In your initial consultation, you're meeting your surgeon and establishing a common goal. The second consultation allows you to go over any further questions you have regarding your individual needs. It permits you to focus on preoperative and postoperative instructions and get a more detailed explanation of the surgery and the recovery. Treatment plans should be formulated for you and your procedure. This second visit will give you the opportunity to go over things with your surgeon and feel comfortable with your decision.

Often the complications of the procedures are glossed over in the first consultation. The second consultation is an opportunity to better go over the risks and complications associated with surgery. General operative complications include anesthetic complications and surgical risks. Procedure-specific complications may also be discussed, including the need for secondary surgeries.

Once again, review your health status with your physician. Don't forget anything. If it takes a while for you to stop bleeding when you cut yourself, that could be critical information. It's important for the surgeon to know you occasionally use an inhaler. They can then give you a "puff" if you start wheezing as you come out of general anesthesia. If you might have had a blood clot after your second pregnancy, further investigation into your family history will be necessary to assess your clotting ability. Don't forget anything, as it may save your life!

Please make sure that the procedure is being performed in a certified operating suite. Certifying and licensing associations exist to inspect surgical suites to ensure they maintain minimum standards to protect the patient. Many of the botched plastic surgery that's performed is by non-qualified providers at noncertified facilities that care little for quality and safety and care only about the bottom line.

A young patient recently died after she succumbed to the anesthesia complication of malignant hyperthermia. Her surgery was performed in an office facility rather than a certified operative suite. Her temperature on arrival to the emergency room was 106 degrees Fahrenheit (normal is 98.6 degrees Fahrenheit). The office surgical suite didn't maintain the antidote Dantrolene in their supplies, so by the time she was transferred to the hospital by ambulance, the antidote was of no benefit. There is safety in numbers, meaning larger surgical facilities have more doctors, nurses, specialized medicines, and equipment available to help handle a problem if it arises.

11. Prepare Yourself for Surgery.

Once the surgical date is set, prepare yourself for the surgery as well as the recovery. If you smoke, please stop well before the surgery. Smoking increases the anesthesia risks as well as surgical complications. The nicotine in cigarettes constricts blood vessels, making them smaller so that not enough blood will flow to the surgical site. A lack of blood flow greatly decreases your healing speed and can lead to skin death, infection, and the potential for poor scarring. Cigarette substitutes containing nicotine aren't a good alternative because the blood vessels are still exposed to a nicotine-rich environment.

Hydrate yourself the day before surgery. You may not have anything to eat or drink the day of surgery and will become dehydrated if you haven't had plenty of fluids the day before surgery. Dehydration destabilizes your cardiovascular system and will increase your risk undergoing general anesthesia. Get plenty of sleep several nights before your surgery as you may not be able to sleep the night before your surgery because of anticipation and excitement. If you're prone to insomnia, discuss this with your surgeon.

Arrange for help with childcare, house cleaning, and laundry. You can better concentrate on what's necessary for a more rapid recovery if you don't have to concern yourself with the needs of others.

12. Adhere to the Postoperative Recovery Path.

The first night after surgery is a critical time as you recover from anesthesia. Have someone stay with you for at least the first 24 hours and preferably 48 hours. Adhere to the postoperative suggestions put forth by your surgeon. Surgeons recommend things that have given their patients the best results. It may be different from what you read about elsewhere, but surgeons have their preference, which you should follow. Don't choose the finest surgeon but then ignore their advice and routine.

Ask questions of the surgeon's staff and schedule follow-up appointments as often as you feel are needed to address your concerns. Some concerns are normal, like swelling on one side if you sleep on that side. But others aren't, such as an infection that induces swelling on one side, and need to be addressed earlier rather than later. Don't neglect to ask any question or to give the office an update on your progress.

Many surgeons see their patients one week after surgery because most complications will manifest at about that time. This includes infections, healing problems, and clots. These are best treated early and aggressively.

13. Allow Adequate Healing to Take Place.

Some patients are upset if things aren't just right at the first post-surgery visit. A lot of initial bad results improve with time and healing. Let the healing process take place, and don't ask for an early revision. Adequate healing cures a lot of problems. An increased risk of complications occurs if corrective operations are performed too soon after the initial surgery. The earliest intervention may be considered at three to four months after surgery, but six to 12 months after is optimum. It may be difficult to wait that long, but healing may correct the concern.

Remember that everyone heals with a scar. Scars are mostly a function of the patient and less of the surgeon. Scars look bad for up to six months. But they will mature and look better with time. Most scar revisions aren't indicated earlier than one year after the incisions have been made. Non-invasive treatments of the scars may be contemplated earlier if indicated. This includes steroid injections and laser therapies.

Most surgeons will say that results are stable at one year after surgery.

Chapter 16

How to Avoid Bad Injections and Laser Treatments

Neuromodulators and fillers should enhance your facial expressions, natural appearance, and your individuality. Lasers and other types of skin-resurfacing devices should do their job and nothing more. Unfortunately, the results are often just the opposite.

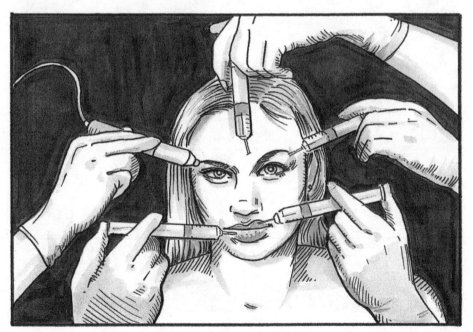

Just as knowing how to protect yourself when choosing a plastic surgeon, this chapter seeks to help you avoid bad results when choosing an injector or laser provider. It's important have work done in an office that specializes in aesthetic procedures and employs professional practitioners. There are many bad and even unethical providers available just waiting for you to walk into their facility. These providers care little for your well-being; they just want your money.

A patient came to see me after getting "free Botox" from a novice injector trying to get some initial experience. Her result was less than flattering.

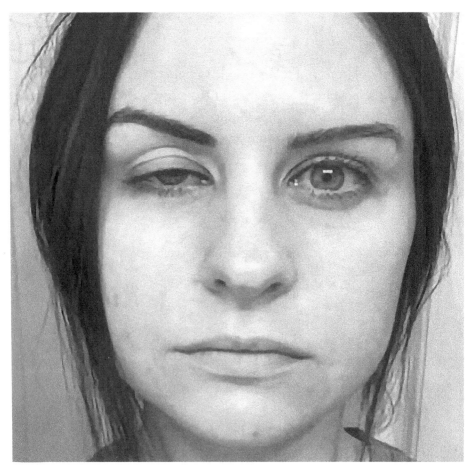

This patient came secondarily after "free" Botox injections by a "resident physician" trying a new neuromodulator.

This hearkens back to the earlier recommendation to avoid free procedures and always know the qualifications and experience of your injector or surgeon. Injections eventually go away but surgical mishaps may last a lifetime.

Below are eight ways to save you from unscrupulous providers. Knowledge is everything, especially when it involves altering your looks.

1. Go to an Injector or Laser Provider with a Good Reputation in the Community.

Get your injectable and laser therapy from a trained professional. Although almost anyone can purchase an injectable, not everyone can inject the filler or neuromodulator appropriately. When you are injecting something below the skin, you have to know what is below the skin and where the important things are located. You want your injector to know exactly what layer they are injecting and know the potentially dangerous areas that contain the blood vessels and nerves. A plastic surgeon or head and neck surgeon will have operated below the skin and knows exactly where the vital structures are located.

2. Give Yourself Plenty of Time to Think about It and Be Comfortable with Your Decision.

While having dental work performed, my patient's dentist said he could make her look younger with some cheek injections delivered while she was anesthetized. She consented and was injected through her mouth into her cheeks at the completion of the dental work. She was left with lumps and bumps asymmetrically in both cheeks. This patient violated this second rule with her rash decision.

3. Make Sure You Know the Injected Material and the Supplier as Well.

My patient had no idea what filler material the dentist injected. Upon questioning the dentist's office, it appeared nothing had been recorded in her chart that would help us. When I asked what the dentist usually uses, the staff confessed that her injection was his first one and that a sales representative left the filler. The information on the filler never came, as the sales representative never returned our calls. We had no idea if the filler would become bigger, how long the filler would last, or if we could dissolve it. We had to wait for months before we could attempt to correct the problem. Many times, it's best to consider the implications of a decision before jumping into unfamiliar territory (especially with an untrained provider).

4. As with Plastic Surgery, Don't Bargain Seek Here Either.

I thought knockoffs were only on handbags and watches on the streets of Manhattan, but they've found their way into providers' offices. If a procedure is deeply discounted, you must exercise caution. The injectable material and lasers are purchased by the provider, who's looking for a return on their investment. Again, if a procedure is deeply discounted, they may be diluting or using misbranded, counterfeit, or knockoff products.

A patient bought some bargain cosmetic filler from an online store using her credit card.[51] A few days later, the filler, shipped from Brazil, arrived. She immediately rushed the package over to her friend who was a nurse but who had no formal training in injecting. The friend injected the woman's cheeks with the Brazilian dermal filler. Within weeks, her cheeks were infected and draining pus from multiple openings through dying skin. Surgery was required to drain the infection and remove as much of the material as possible. Examination of the material showed it to be glass or fiberglass. When the Brazilian company was contacted, they responded that her problems "had nothing to do with the product but with the injection procedure." Sadly, her problems were the result of the material *and* the injector.

Between 2015 and 2019, an unlicensed "injector" defrauded her customers by selling counterfeit medical devices.[52] These devices were foreign-made fillers that weren't approved by the FDA for use in the US. The injector shipped the filler through her retail company and then used the United States Postal Service to ship the counterfeit products to her customers. This case was investigated by the FDA, the United States Postal Inspection Service, and the Department of Homeland Security.

In 2020, the US Customs and Border Protection Agency seized six shipments of prohibited cosmetic injection material including dermal fillers and counterfeit Botox. The shipments were purchased online from various countries but were all addressed to private residences in the US. The Customs Border Protection warned that the materials were manufactured in unregulated facilities with substandard ingredients and no quality controls. The seizure was executed to assure the health and safety of US citizens.[53]

5. Ask about the Qualifications of the Injector or the Person Performing the Laser Therapy and Make Sure You're Comfortable with Them.

When performing Botox injections, subtleties count, and the improvements seen with qualified injectors are amazing. The injection sites and the injection amounts are only recommendations by the manufacturer. A "cookbook" approach to Botox injections doesn't always fit every person and an experienced injector appreciates the differences. The subtleties of injecting just a little bit higher, a little bit lower, a little bit deeper, a little bit shallower, or with a little less or more toxin can make all the difference.

I watch and analyze each patient's face, as I engage in small talk, just to see how their muscles are moving. It can be different every time the patient visits. The Botox dosage and injection locations may need to be changed. Doing it the same way at each and every visit may not be appropriate.

We also know that the face changes with long-term neuromodulator use. The injected muscles become weaker, forcing other muscle groups to take over. Because of this muscle recruitment, facial expressions can become weird. For example, if the muscles between the eyebrows no longer work, the muscles of the nose may take over resulting in deep "bunny lines" across the top of the nose between the eyes. These will then require correction as well.

The greatest problem with any injectable is using *too much*. Using too much neuromodulator can paralyze the face. Too much filler can make the person look inflated and strange. Injections should be performed judicially because most injectable material can't be reversed. If necessary, more can always be added later.

Knowing how your injector was trained is critical to the outcome you receive. They need to be well trained and not someone the staff says does "hundreds of these a year." The bonus to knowing their background is that you can gain a sense of comfort knowing you're in capable hands.

6. Make Sure Clear Instructions Are Received That Explain How to Care for Your Skin after a Laser Treatment.

Post-laser care of the skin is important and something frequently not addressed by providers. An ablative laser treatment leaves the skin raw. Poor or nonexistent care after the laser procedure will leave the patient with post-inflammatory dark areas or even scars. Many noncertified providers don't understand wound healing and don't give appropriate post-laser skin care instructions to prevent complications.

If you have a laser treatment, ask what skin care products are recommended to prevent unwanted brown pigmentation and scarring, keep the skin hydrated, and protect the compromised skin from sun damage.

7. Ask What the Policies Are if You Receive an Unexpected Result.

It's better to know what the facility policy is if you receive a bad result *before* you undergo treatment. If a less skilled provider does the initial treatment and causes the problem, you probably don't want them to do the corrective intervention.

8. Set Appropriate Expectations.

Don't expect a large improvement with less-invasive procedures. Minimally invasive procedures are oversold to people hungry for procedures with no downtime. These procedures rarely deliver as promised and can even be misused to the point of injury to the patient. Many physicians advertise lesser procedures to get patients into their office only to tell the patient that they need a more invasive and expensive procedure. Or worse, they perform the less-invasive procedure only to recommend the more expensive procedure after the initial result isn't what the patient expected.

Be concerned if you're shown pictures of noninvasive procedures and think, "How did that happen?" or "No way!" Those striking results can only be from surgery. Nothing removes wrinkles, tightens the skin, and repositions dropped structures like surgery. Even with all the advances made in skin care, chemical peels, lasers, heating and cooling devices, and injectables (fillers and neuromodulators), none of these less-invasive techniques will give you a result comparable to a forehead lift, an eyelid surgery, a facelift, or a neck lift.

Only surgery gives you the "drop-dead great result" which will make people exclaim, "*You look marvelous!*"

Afterword

P lastic surgery doesn't need to be bad. After reading this book, you should now understand what causes bad plastic surgery and, even better, know how to avoid those bad plastic surgery mistakes. Don't be surprised if, after all you've learned, you'll now see why there is "sooo much bad plastic surgery" out there as you look at people around you.

With good plastic surgery, you should look at your face and body in a mirror and feel confident and beautiful. People should look at you after a plastic surgery procedure and think, "Boy, they look great!" and not, "Oh no, look what they had done." Good plastic surgery emphasizes and corrects in a natural, flattering way. Plastic surgery, done well, means your classmates at your next reunion will say, "You look as good today as you did at graduation thirty years ago."

While plastic surgery is all about the outward appearance, you might be surprised to find that you think differently about yourself in the same way as a former patient confided to me: "At sixty-six, I feel better about myself than I did when I was twenty or thirty years old. I feel more like a woman, and I'm now empowered to care about and for myself."

Post-plastic surgery, you'll find yourself embracing the positive changes of aesthetic refinements, living a better quality of life, feeling more personal confidence, and enjoying your improved interpersonal relationships. You'll still be you, only better.

And please remember, plastic surgery shouldn't scream; it should whisper!

About the Author

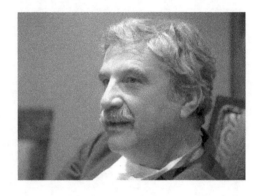

D r. Thomas J. Francel, MD, is a highly respected, board-certified plastic surgeon with an established private practice in St. Louis for over 30 years. He completed his surgical residency at Harvard Surgical Services and furthered his specialty in plastic surgery at Johns Hopkins Hospital. His contributions to medical literature include 22 peer-reviewed articles and 19 book chapters in various surgical journals. He is a sought-after speaker and educator, having presented his knowledge and techniques at over 20 national and international plastic surgery conferences. In 1999, he gained national recognition when he was interviewed by ABC's *20/20*, where he shed light on the causes and treatments of severe post-surgical infections.

Abbreviations

ABCS: American Board of Cosmetic Surgery
ABMS: American Board of Medical Specialties
ABPS: American Board of Plastic Surgery
ACGME: Accreditation Council for Graduate Medical Education
ASAPS: American Society of Aesthetic Plastic Surgeons
ASPS: American Society of Plastic Surgeons
BDD: Body Dysmorphic Disorder
ENT: Ear, Nose, and Throat
FDA: Food and Drug Administration
FOMO: Fear of Missing Out
IPL: Intense pulse light
MBC: Medical Board of California
OCD: Obsessive-compulsive disorder
OMF: Oral Maxillofacial
OR: Operating room
PIP: Poly Implant Prostheses
RF: Radio-frequency
ROI: Return on investment
SEO: Search engine optimization
WHR: Waist-to-hips ratio

Endnotes

Chapter 3

1 Marquardt, Stephen, "Method and Apparatus for Analyzing Facial Configurations and Components," US Patent 5,659,625, filed May 23, 1994, and issued August 19,1997.

2 Daily Mail Reporter, "Bat Brows and Trout Pouts: When Surgery Goes Wrong," Daily Mail, September 2, 2009, Femail, https://www.dailymail.co.uk/femail/beauty/article-1210563/Bat-brows-trout-pouts-When-surgery-goes-wrong.html.

Chapter 4

3 "2020 Plastic Surgery Statistic Report," *American Society of Plastic Surgery*, https://www.plasticsurgery.org/documents/News/Statistics/2020/plastic-surgery-statistics-full-report-2020.pdf.

4 Sarwer, DB PhD, Gibbons, LM, Magee L, et al., "A Prospective, Multi-Site Investigation of Patient Satisfaction and Psychosocial Status Following Cosmetic Surgery," *Aesthetic Surgery Journal*, 2005;25: 263-269.

5 Reilly, MJ, Tomsic, JA, Fernandez SJ, Davison, SP, "Effect of Facial rejuvenation Surgery on Perceived Attractiveness, Femininity, and Personality," *JAMA Facial Plastic Surgery*, 2015;17: 202-207.

6 Herrick, D, PhD, National Center for Policy Analysis. AAPS News, September 2013.

7 Gordan, C, DO, Pryor, L, MD, Afifi, A MD, et al, "Cosmetic Surgery Volume and Its Correlation with the Major US Stock Market Indices," *Aesthetic Surgery Journal*, 2010; 30: 470-475.

8 See note 1 above.

9   See note 1 above.

Chapter 6

10   Associated Press, "U.S. Warns Doctors on Canadian Botox," *CBC News*, December 24, 2012, Health, https://www.cbc.ca/news/health/u-s-warns-doctors-on-canadian-botox-1.1292410.

11   "FDA Warns About Counterfeit Botox," *CBS News*, April 17, 2015, https://www.cbsnews.com/news/fda-warns-about-counterfeit-botox/.

12   Dorfman RG, Purnell C, Qiu C, et al., "Happy and Unhappy Patients: A Quantitative Analysis of Online Plastic Surgeon Reviews for Breast Augmentation," *Plastic and Reconstructive Surgery*, May 2018, 141 p 663-673e.

Chapter 7

13   Bone, J. The Curse of Beauty: The Scandalous and Tragic Life of Audrey Munson, America's First Supermodel, Regan Arts, 2017.

Chapter 8

14   "2018 Plastic Surgery Statistic Report," American Society of Plastic Surgery, https://www.plasticsurgery.org/documents/News/Statistics/2018/plastic-surgery-statistics-full-report-2018.pdf.

15   Gorney, M, Martello, J, "Patient Selection Criteria," Clinical Plastic Surgery, 1999;26:37-40.

Chapter 10

16   Shah, A MD, Patel, A MD, MBA, Smetona, J, MD, Rohrich, R MD, "Public Perception of Cosmetic Surgeons versus Plastic Surgeons: Increasing Transparency to Educate Patients," Plastic Reconstructive Surgery, 139: 544e, 2017.

17   Erdely, SR., "Nipped, Tucked, and Wide Awake?" *Self Magazine,* January 2011.

18   "About ABMS," *American Board of Medical Specialties*, https://abms. org/about-abms/.

19   "24 Member Boards," *American Board of Medical Specialties*, https:// abms.org/member-boards/.

20   Press Release, *PR Newswire*, https://www.prnewswire.com/news-releases/federal-court-upholds-the-right-of-plastic-surgeons-to-promote-abps-board-certification-228371301.html.

21   Press Release, "The Aesthetic Society Congratulates the Utah Plastic Surgery Society For Taking A Stand," *Cosmetic Surgery Associates*, https://cosmeticplastics.com/cosmetic-surgery-2/aesthetic-society-congratulates-utah-plastic-surgery-society-stand/.

22   Jordan, SW MD, Mioton, LM BS, Smetona, J BA, BS, et al., "An Analysis of 10,356 Patients from the American College of Surgeons National Surgical Quality Improvement Program Database," *Plastic and Reconstructive Surgery*, 2013:131(4):763-773.

23   Campbell, A JD, Cloud, L JD, Ghorashi, A JD, "Office Based Surgery Laws," *The Policy Surveillance Program at Temple University Beasley School of Law*, August 2016.

24   "Selected Provisions of Office Based Surgery Statutes, Regulations, Policies, and Guidelines," *American Society of Plastic Surgeons,* April 2014.

25   Jalian, HR. MD, Jalian, CA, JD, Avram, MM. MD, JD, "Increased Risk of Litigation Associated with Laser Surgery by Non-Physician Operators," *JAMA Dermatology*, 2014:150(4): 407–4011.

26   O'Donnell, Jayne, "Lack of training can be deadly in cosmetic surgery," *ABC News*, September 13, 2011, https://abcnews.go.com/Business/lack-training-deadly-cosmetic-surgery/story?id=14514234.

27   Custom, Lisa, "Two Women Dead After Liposuction, Police Say," *Courthouse News Service*, August 9, 2013, https://www.courthousenews.com/two-women-dead-afterliposuction-police-say/.

28   Hahn, Valerie Schremp, "Death of St. Louis County Woman Highlights Risks of Illegal Buttocks Injections," *STL Today*,

August 6, 2015, https://www.stltoday.com/news/local/crime-and-courts/death-of-st-louis-county-woman-highlights-risks-of-illegal-buttocks-injections/article_eaf694b3-a4af-51de-8fbd-77bc522895e0.html.

29 "'Dr Lipjob' Ordered to Stop Injecting Botox, Impersonating Doctor," *CBC News*, November 21, 2018, https://www.cbc.ca/news/canada/british-columbia/dr-lipjob-ordered-to-stop-injecting-botox-impersonating-doctor-1.4635618

30 Ovalle, David, "The Penis and Butt Surgeries Went Way Wrong. And a Fake Doctor Will Pay for It," Miami Herald, October 2, 2017, https://www.miamiherald.com/news/local/crime/article176571176.html.

31 Rocha, Veronica, "A Woman Got 'Lamb Fat' Injected into Her Buttocks; Now She Needs Major Reconstructive Surgery," *LA Times* June 28, 2017, https://www.latimes.com/local/lanow/la-me-ln-lambs-fat-buttocks-injections-charges-20170628-htmlstory.html.

32 Associated Press, "NJ Woman Pleads Guilty in Man's Death After Penis Enlargement," *NBC New York,* September 9, 2015, https://www.nbcnewyork.com/news/local/woman-charge-man-death-silicone-injection-penis-kasia-rivera/2010011/#:~:text=A%20New%20Jersey%20woman%20has,%2C%20according%20to%20NJ.com.

33 Liston, Barbara, "Man Charged with Manslaughter in Florida Butt-Injection Case," *Reuters Health News*, July 27, 2012, https://br.reuters.com/article/oukoe-uk-usa-crime-butt-injection/man-charged-with-manslaughter-in-florida-butt-injection-case-idUKBRE86Q0H220120727.

34 "The FDA Requests Allergan Voluntarily Recall Natrelle BIOCELL Textured Breast Implants and Tissue Expanders from the Market to Protect Patients," *FDA Safety Communication*, June 1, 2020, https://www.fda.gov/medical-devices/safety-communications/fda-requests-allergan-voluntarily-recall-natrelle-biocell-textured-breast-implants-and-tissue.

Chapter 11

35 Associated Press, "Usher's Wife Checks Out of Brazilian Hospital," *Deseret News*, February 18, 2009, https://www.deseret.com/2009/2/18/20302658/usher-s-wife-checks-out-of-brazil-hospital.

36 Hopkins, Anna, "Plastic Surgeon Warns Against 'Medical Tourism' After Third Plastic Surgery-Related Death in Dominican Republic," *Fox News*, July 11, 2019, Dominican Republic, https://www.foxnews.com/health/plastic-surgeon-dominican-republic-deaths.

37 Schnabel, D, Esposito, DH, Gaines J. Multistate, "US Outbreak of Rapidly Growing Mycobacterial Infections Associated with Medical Tourism to the Dominican Republic, 2013-2014," *Emerging Infectious Diseases*, 2016:22 (8) 1340-1347.

38 Farid, M, Nikkhah, D, Little, M., "Complications of Plastic Surgery Abroad—Cost Analysis and Patient Perception," *PRS Global Open*, 2019:7:e2281.

Chapter 12

39 Press Release, "Attorney General Cuomo Secures Settlement with Plastic Surgery Franchise That Flooded Internet with False Positive Reviews," New York State Office of the Attorney General, July 14, 2009, https://ag.ny.gov/press-release/2009/attorney-general-cuomo-secures-settlement-plastic-surgery-franchise-flooded.

40 Ibid.

41 Swift, A., "Americans Say Social Media Have Little Sway on Purchases," Gallup Poll, published June 23, 2014.

42 Zahedi, SZ, Hancock E, Hameed S, et.al., "Social Media's Influence on Breast Augmentation," Aesthetic Surgery Journal, 2020;40: 917-925.

Chapter 13

43   Parina, R, Chang, D, Sead, AN, et.al., "Quality and Safety Outcomes of Ambulatory Plastic Surgery Facilities in California," *Plastic and Reconstructive Surgery*, 2015:135:791-797.

Chapter 14

44   Gusenoff JA, Coon D, Nayer H, et al., "Medial Thigh Lift in the Massive Weight Loss Population, Outcomes and Complications," Plastic and Reconstructive Surgery, 2015;135:98-106.

45   Forster, NA, Kunzi W, Giovanoli, P., "The Reoperation Cascade After Breast Augmentation with Implants: What the Patient Needs to Know," Journal of Plastic, Reconstructive and Aesthetic Surgery, 2013; 66: 313-322.

Chapter 15

46   Mitchell, Kirk, "Fake Denver doctor charged with sexual assault and criminal impersonation," Denver Post, August 23, 2016, News: Crime and Public Safety, https://www.denverpost.com/2016/08/23/fake-denver-doctor-charged-sexual-assault-criminal-impersonation/.

47   Cary Grant in *North by Northwest,* MGM, 1959.

48   Chen, K MD, Congiusta, S RN, Nash, IS MD, et al., "Factors Influencing Patient Satisfaction in Plastic Surgery: A Nationwide Analysis," Plastic and Reconstructive Surgery, 2018, 142:820-825.

49   Ibid.

50   Rivers, J, Frankel, V., *Men Are Stupid…And They Like Big Boobs*, New York: Pocket Books, December 2009.

Chapter 16

51   Tamura, T, Lah, K., "DIY Plastic Surgery Leads to Horrific Injuries," *The Baltimore Times*, July 7, 2014.

52   Staff, "Merrillville Woman Faces Charges for Allegedly Importing Fraudulent Medical Devices: U.S. Attorney," Chicago Post Tribune, June 18, 2020, Suburbs, https://www.chicagotribune.com/

suburbs/post-tribune/ct-ptb-merrillville-woman-indicted-st-0619-20200618-d4zwclekgzb5tpzz2vdsn2ohna-story.html.

53   Mitchell, Madeline, "US Customs: Over $35,000 Worth of Counterfeit Botox Seized in Cincinnati," *The Cincinnati Enquirer*, August 27, 2020, News, https://www.cincinnati.com/story/news/2020/08/27/u-s-customs-over-35-000-worth-counterfeit-botox-seized-cincinnati/5646210002/.

A free ebook edition
is available with the
purchase of this book.

To claim your free ebook edition:

1. Visit MorganJamesBOGO.com
2. Sign your name CLEARLY in the space
3. Complete the form and submit a photo of the entire copyright page
4. You or your friend can download the ebook to your preferred device

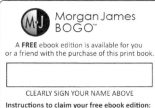

Morgan James
BOGO™

A **FREE** ebook edition is available for you or a friend with the purchase of this print book.

CLEARLY SIGN YOUR NAME ABOVE

Instructions to claim your free ebook edition:
1. Visit MorganJamesBOGO.com
2. Sign your name CLEARLY in the space above
3. Complete the form and submit a photo of this entire page
4. You or your friend can download the ebook to your preferred device

Print & Digital Together Forever.

Snap a photo

Free ebook

Read anywhere

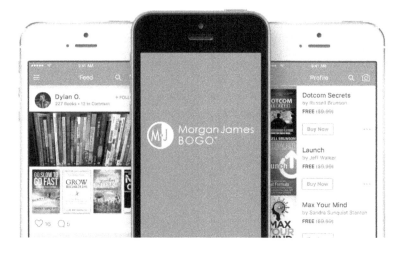

Printed in the USA
CPSIA information can be obtained
at www.ICGtesting.com
JSHW022150061124
73101JS00008B/217